FAITH, LOVE, AND APPLESAUCE

Facing Childhood Leukemia Head-on, and Coming Out the Otherside.

Kimberly Koegel

CONTENTS

Hi my name is Taylor Koegel and this book is composed of daily journals that my mom wrote every day during my treatment process. For 2 years, 3-5 years old, I went through treatment for childhood leukemia. Now I am 16 years old and a grateful survivor with the very blessed opportunity to share my story knowing that friends I had through treatment don't have the same opportunity. I would like to dedicate this to the friends I met at Shands, my family, my friends, and the doctors who saved my life (and the thought of no more applesauce). Thank you.

JANUARY 23, 2007

Thank you for visiting Taylor's site and checking in on her progress. She was diagnosed with Leukemia (ALL) Pre-B on January 20, 2007 and completed her treatments on March 22, 2009. Thank you everyone for your love and support, and for your web site postings. It all means so much.

So that everyone understands how this diagnosis came about, I'll give you some history of the past week. This started on Thursday (January 18th) when her school called to tell us that she was falling asleep during circle time and had a fever of 102 degrees. We went and picked her up, tried to treat with Tylenol and rest throughout the day, but her fever continued to climb until it reached 104.6. That prompted a visit to urgent care that night, during which they took a blood sample (because they couldn't identify the root cause of her fever, which was concerning to them). Later that night, the pediatrician on call for our pediatrician's office contacted me and let me know that there were some concerns about the bloodwork, and that we needed to be at our doctor's office first thing Friday morning. While the call concerned me, I had no idea what was in store. When we arrived at Dr. Elzie's office on Friday morning, and he was made aware of the situation and the lab results, he quickly brought us back to an exam room, starting checking her, and explained to us the severity of her condition. He explained that it was indicative of leukemia, and that we needed to go to Shands Children Hospital in order to meet with specialists who could do further tests to confirm or rule out that diagnosis. He explained to us that Taylor would need to be taken to Shands in an ambulance that day, but prior to going, she would need to be admitted into our local hospital to do additional assessments to confirm whether or not she would need a blood transfusion prior to being sent to Shands. We ended up at Shands later on Friday evening, and have been submerged in this ever since. The official diagnosis came Saturday night after her oncologist completed a bone marrow biopsy. This test allowed him to confirm both that it was leukemia, as well as the specific type: Acute Lymphoblastic Leukemia (ALL). On Sunday, there was a subsequent bone marrow biopsy done as well as a spinal tap- also called a lumbar puncture (LP). The LP was completed for 2 reasons: (1) to obtain and test a sample of spinal fluid to identify if the cancer had spread to her brain, and (2) to inject chemotherapy treatment into her spinal fluid so that they could treat any potential cancer cells that may have formed in the brain already. We received very good news yesterday (Monday) that her LP fluid came back clear, meaning that there were no cancer cells in her brain. We still have additional genetic mapping tests that will be done this week that will help finalize the diagnosis as well as the course of her treatment, and there is definitely a lot of literature for us to read, but no one can convince us of anything but a full recovery. She is a fighter (as she has definitely proved to the nurses and doctors today via some of her persistent outbursts related to the steroid treatments), and we know that her strong will and spirit will be that much more important as treatment continues.

Our intent is to update this site frequently and let people know the latest...it is hard to be able to return all of our phone messages, but please know that we are so appreciative of the phone calls, the cards, and your prayers. With your love and support, we will all be able to get through this and see her through to recovery.

Love, Rob, Kim, Taylor and Alex

January 23, 2007

As I am writing this, Taylor is finishing up Day 3 of her treatment for Leukemia (ALL) Pre- B. There is a 29-day induction period of treatment, and we are taking it one step at a time. She is happy, scared, angry, frustrated- a range of emotions. It is hard to say that there are 'good days and bad days' so far...there are instead 'good hours and bad hours.'

Her treatment to date has included both chemotherapy treatments as well as steroid medications- some of which cause dramatic mood swings. While this is trying on her daddy and me, we know that the medicine is causing this to happen, and that the combination of the side effects and her own fears about what is going on result in her outbursts.

We can't say enough about the doctors, nurses, and staff at Shands. We have met with 'Child's Life' coordinators who manage the 'Play room ' activities and also focus on distraction techniques for the kids. This gives Taylor a chance to do some of the things she loves most- draw, play with Play-doh, play with toys and puzzles, and drive a car up and down the halls of the hospital.

She is getting used to her 'buddy' (i.e., her PICC line) that is attached to her arm. This allows the nurses to draw blood samples without having to poke her every few hours. This also allows them to just hook up any sort of IV fluids or antibiotics that she needs.

Taylor is also meeting other kids that are in her situation. I think that makes the greatest impact on her, and makes her feel like there are other kids just like her close by. The kids really help each other out. On our second day here, one of the kids saw that she was having a hard time with her IV (this was prior to her PICC line being put in), and he explained to her that it would be easier for her once her PICC line was in.

Another little girl (Taylor's age) is a month into treatment, and has lost her hair. Taylor and her played yesterday, and we talked about how Zoe's hair was getting shorter, and that it was okay. That also prompted a hair styling session tonight with Taylor, Mommy, and Daddy. We let Taylor snip some of our hair off, and we snipped a little bit of length off of hers...we'll play 'hair salon' as she wants to so that it is less traumatic (to the extent possible) when she loses all of her hair over the next couple of weeks.

Taylor also has a 'chemo duck' stuffed animal that one of the counselors gave us yesterday. They also gave us a child's medical kit so that we can help do medical role playing with Taylor. Chemo duck has a port line (just like Taylor will have), and he wears a bandana because his hair isn't there anymore. Taylor has taken to carrying him around, and we did some role playing tonight about the shots she will be getting tomorrow as part of her treatment.

Well, with that, I am signing off for the night. She is resting peacefully right now, and with the exception of vital sign checks, should not have to be woken up tonight for anything specific. Love to everyone, and thanks for your messages today.

January 24, 2007

Thank you to everyone for your messages. It brings smiles and tears of appreciation for Rob and I to know that so many people are thinking of Taylor and helping us get through this.

Thank you for the beautiful flowers, balloons, and gifts that people are sending....one item that I wasn't aware of is that fresh flowers and latex balloons cannot be kept in our room. They are keeping the nurse's station very pretty though, and we go out to visit them often.

Here are some updates from today about Miss Taylor: She is on Day 4 of her treatment. Today was an anxious day because she was getting a 2 shot regimen of a drug called PEG

Asparaginase. It is given by a shot into her leg. As you can imagine, we looked to the counselors and nurses here to help us prepare her for this, as this particular shot can be painful. Taylor did great. We told her to scream as loud as she wanted to. And she did, but then she was fine. Looking at the roadmap of treatment she has during the induction period, that should be the only dose of Asparaginase on the schedule. So we are thankful for that. We are trying to take lots of walks (or hop like a bunny down the hall) so that we keep our muscles strong. One of the side effects of one of the chemo drugs can be weakening of her muscles. She has been good about taking walks, but then we also carry her around the halls when she starts to get cabin fever.

Taylor told us today that if she doesn't have hair, she won't have to wash it anymore. It was interesting, because the comment came out of nowhere- we weren't even talking about her hair at the time...so it is something for Rob and I to be aware of...that she is constantly listening to everything we hear and say, and that she is contemplating what that means to her.

Taylor wants to type some letters for everyone. Here they are! dmmmmmmmmmmmmmmmmmmmmmmmmmfcd kj B

We love you and will send more updates soon.

January 25, 2007

Thank you, thank you, thank you for everything people are doing for us. The cards, pictures, treats for Taylor, toiletries, everything has just overwhelmed us with how much she is loved....I could say thank you a million times, and never be able to thank everyone enough. I did want to let everyone know that Godby High School is sponsoring a 'Relay for Life' Event in March this year (this is associated with the American Cancer Society). My sister Debbie teaches at Godby, and has been part of this event over the past few years, and has been on a planning committee for it this year. Who knew that this event would mean even that much more to us this year...When I get back to Tallahassee, I would like to get a team established and walk for Taylor...and for all of the others battling this awful disease. There is also a little boy at Taylor's school who was diagnosed just 2 days ahead of her, so they are fighting this together. When we do get back to Tallahassee, I plan to work with my sister to understand how to get signed up and continue raising money for the event in March. I think this is a wonderful event, and sadly, I know that we all have been impacted at some point in our lives by knowing someone that has had to battle cancer.

Godby is having a kick-off event tonight at their media center at 6 p.m. If you are interested in participating, I'd encourage you to attend and find out more tonight. I will ask my sister if there is an e-mail address or contact info for folks that have more questions about the event, but she did say to feel free to just show up tonight (Thursday, 1/25). It is just a very timely event with everything going on at the moment...

We send our love to everyone. We did have kind of an interesting night...the floor above us had a flood, and so we had to quickly change hospital rooms around 11:00 p.m. last night. One thing it did force us to do was downsize a bit from the toys we had in the room and get some of them moved to the minivan. I am telling myself that we are just starting to pack early....hopeful for a discharge from the hospital in the next couple of days. We will still need to be within 20 minutes of the hospital for the remainder of her induction period (approximately the next month), but it will be a change of scenery for her.

She had a very restful night, and today's medicine regimen should just be the steroid treatment. We have been experimenting with different coping mechanisms (suggestions provided by the nurses, doctors, counselors) to help Taylor deal with her frustrations some more. And we are on Day 5...so we are getting closer to some key milestones in her recovery. Day 8 is our next key milestone. I will read through the documentation we have so that I can explain more about that later and the procedures that will be done to confirm the percentage of leukemia cells still in her body...but that is a key milestone date for us.

Taylor's daddy gave her a cute haircut last night. I guess you could call it a 'bob' style...while I think he should still keep his day job, she is very pleased with her new haircut. We let her snip some more hair from each of us as well. I saved a pretty lock of her hair though. We are trying as best as we can to help her understand that having no hair will be fine. She is just excited that she won't have to wash it for a period of time. She says that the soap won't get in her eyes now.

January 25, 2007

Just time for a quick update- as I have very good news. We are packing up her hospital room for our planned departure tomorrow! The doctors feel that she is stable enough to leave the hospital on oral medications (i.e., she doesn't have to have things through an IV for now), and we can move to an off-site apartment for the next 3 weeks. We have to be within 20 minutes of the hospital in case she gets a fever over 100.4 degrees, and needs to be readmitted. Those out there with kids know that 100.4 doesn't sound very high, so we will be watching her very closely! We will still be going to the hospital on a regular basis for clinical visits and dosages of IV medicine, but Rob and I will also be administering oral medications at the apartment. We are hopeful that the remainder of the induction period will go fine, and are praying about the outcome of Day 8 (which Day 8 is technically Sunday, so we won't have the procedure typically done on Day 8 until Day 9). On Day 9 (next Monday), she will have another lumbar puncture procedure (LP) and bone marrow biopsy which will help assess her leukemia counts. That is a big day for Taylor, as it will give us an idea of how the treatment is progressing. We will send more later. Little Taylor is sleeping right now, so we need to pack up...love to everyone.

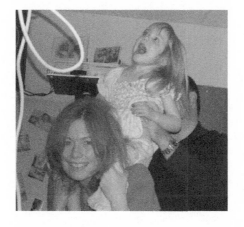

FROM HOSPITAL
TO HOTEL

January 26, 2007

Taylor was discharged today, and we are now moved into our 'new hotel' as we are calling it for Taylor. Several of you have asked for the new address, and I will update it on the website as well, but here it is:

Residence Inn by Marriott, Attn: Rob and Kim Koegel 4001 SW 13th Street
Gainesville, FL 32608

Every day I will start off with saying 'Thank you,' because as we've mentioned before, there are no words to describe how much we appreciate everyone's support. Tallahassee Fire Department, Leon County EMS, fire/rescue from around the State, Accenture, Scottsdale Academy and families- just to name a few- you guys have been amazing. Friends and family, and people who we may have never met are putting her on prayer chains, and we really believe these prayers are making a difference.

Taylor loves the pretty cards and drawings that people are sending. We have decorated the hotel with pictures, cards and her personal things so that she can feel as much at home as possible.

A friend sent us 2 'Live Strong' bracelets today and I started crying. We're wearing them, and will continue to. Robbie and I are both trying to understand how and why this happened, and we know there is a plan, but are just hoping someday to understand the purpose. Other than her mood swings from the medicines she is on, she still seems like our happy little girl. The doctors have explained that her strength will start to go down as the chemotherapy continues, and that's when we will really see the difference in our little Taylor. It seems backwards in a way- that getting better means having to get worse first.

Robbie is going to be headed out soon to the pharmacy to pick up her various medications. She has been getting better about taking them, but she says they still taste 'spicy and yucky.' I told her that they probably do, but they will help make her cancer germs go away.

Little sister Alex is coming to visit this weekend, so Taylor is happy. We have so appreciated the visits from family and friends. Some visits have had to be short in order to accommodate for her needs for rest, so we appreciate the understanding. As we get further into her treatment, we'll have a better feel for when she can have longer visits. Everyone has been good about wearing masks and using a lot of Purell. I was joking the other day that I would love to be the Shands' rep for Purell....it is everywhere! Alrighty, we are signing off for now. Miss Taylor is waking up from a nap. Love to all...

January 27, 2007

Day 7 of treatment....but a great morning for Taylor, as she woke up in the 'new hotel' as opposed to the hospital. It is amazing what an impact the change of environment has had on her today. She has had the opportunity to go spend time outside without a mask, and that has made her happy. What made her happiest of all was seeing Little Alex today. Grandma, Grandpa, Aunt Debbie and Alex came to visit today. When they got here, we found a park nearby and had a picnic outside. There weren't any other people around, so Taylor was able to roam freely without a mask and enjoy some outside air. The park was very close to our hotel, so as soon as she felt tired, we were able to be back in our room within just a few minutes. It brought tears to my eyes when she first saw Alex and Alex saw her. Debbie pulled Alex out of the car, and Alex started literally screaming 'Tay Tay, Tay, Tay' (her name for Taylor). And Taylor was basically jumping out of my arms to get to Alex. Even at such a young age, siblings can have such a bond...I hope they continue to be close. I know I wouldn't be getting through this without my sister's support.

We did make a quick visit to the hospital today, but not for anything too concerning. We weren't able to effectively flush one of her PICC line tubes (I'm sure there is a more technical name, but remember who is writing this), so we called the Pediatrics floor to understand if we needed to bring her in so they could do it. They had us come up, and said that there was just something small blocking it, but it was something they could fix pretty quickly. We were in and out within 15 minutes. She will go back for an overnight stay on Sunday night (in preparation for her biopsy and lumbar puncture on Monday). Her platelets are low, so they will need to give her platelets tomorrow night so she can have the procedure on Monday.

On a different front, Rob is teaching me a lot about how to draw up her medicine in the right amounts and to feel comfortable giving all of the doses. I know he will have me feeling comfortable with flushing out her PICC line before I know it.

Rob and I are very anxious about her procedure on Monday. It will give us a sense of the percentage of leukemia cells still in her body. While we are refusing to tell ourselves that anything but a full recovery will happen, there is always the concern that she will not be in remission by the end of the induction period. I know it seems quick to consider remission at the end of a 29-day period, but it is what the doctors expect according to the standard treatment schedule. I don't want to focus on any negative thoughts, so we will just try to stay positive, and hope for a good outcome from Monday's procedure.

The mood swings were less frequent today- we are attributing that to the change of scenery and more freedom to roam at the 'new hotel.' We have actually set up little 'centers' for her like she has at school. She is excited about that. At school, she tells me that one of her favorite centers is 'Home Living,' so we set up a home living center with her games and dress up clothes. She also has a 'Library' center with all of her books, and an 'Arts and Crafts' center with her Play-Doh, coloring books, stamps, and paints. While it will be impossible to simulate normal life, it is our 'new normal.' Kathy, a friend of the family whose son is battling Leukemia, told me that term last week, and I think it is appropriate. Life will not be normal now, but we can try to accept the 'new normal' to the extent possible.

Thanks for all of the updates to the guestbook. Your words and updates mean a lot to us. As soon as we have an update on the outcome of her procedure on Monday, I will get it out to everyone via the website....

January 29, 2007

Day 9- and a big day in terms of procedures. Taylor had a lumbar puncture (LP) today and a bone marrow biopsy. The results will not be back until Wednesday because the doctors have to do some additional analysis of it to accurately know the percentage of leukemia lymphoblasts that still exist in her body. The goal is to have less than 4%. It is not common for this to happen by Day 8 /9, which is why there is a subsequent LP scheduled for Day 14 as part of the standard protocol. By Day 14, and no later than Day 29, the doctors expect this to happen. Our goal is that by Day 29, Taylor is in RER (Rapid Early Remission). As soon as we have the results from today's procedure, I will let everyone know.

One promising thing that the Dr. mentioned today was that Taylor's white cells and platelets were at a higher level than expected when they drew blood last night. The reason that we had to admit Taylor to the hospital last night was so she could have platelets prior to the procedure today. When she left the hospital on Friday, her platelets were at 22 (the scale they use to measure the platelet levels). They won't do this procedure with platelets less than 40; hence, the reason for giving her platelets Sunday night. Prior to giving her the platelets Sunday night, they drew blood for labs, and her platelets had gone from 22 - 29 since Friday. Her white cell count was also up. The doctor said that this is a positive sign that she seems to be responding well to the treatment. This doesn't change the standard course, as the protocol is clear about which treatments / medicines which will be given on each day. But, it is a glimmer of hope that Rob and I were happy to hear as we are in the midst of all of this.

Today was probably one of the toughest days to date with regard to side effects from the treatments. Taylor is very frustrated, and the steroids make her act out just terribly. I am so thankful that Robbie and I can be here supporting each other. We have to constantly remind ourselves that the medicine is causing her to act this way. It is not the Taylor we know.

On a slightly lighter side, Taylor has a non-stop appetite. There is no breakfast, lunch, and dinner. It is one continuous meal. She woke up this morning and asked for a chicken quesadilla, a chicken leg, cheese pizza, grilled cheese, chicken nuggets, french fries, Doritos, pink lemonade, and chocolate pudding. That was not her request for the day- it was instead her request for breakfast. The doctors keep telling us to feed her whatever she is craving. The interesting thing is that she finishes the majority of what she asks for. I don't know where she puts it all. Although, as you can imagine, her tummy is bothering her from time to time, but from everyone we've talked to, they say that the steroids are giving her an appetite, she needs to eat, and we need to keep on providing the food. I have had to get used to being okay with her eating chocolate pudding for breakfast, but it is a minor concession in light of the situation.

Well, I better run. Miss Taylor would like some more Cheez-It crackers, and Rob is out picking up some rice for her. Thank you everyone for your postings. We try to read them every night. It means so much to hear from everyone.

Love, Kim and Rob

January 30, 2007

Thank you so much to everyone for everything you are doing. We love reading Taylor the cards that come in the mail each day, she loves looking at all of the pictures, and we are very appreciative of the various ways that people are helping to alleviate day to day costs. Please know that we will be forever appreciative. And thank you for all of your postings...please keep them coming as they are something that really keep us going.

Day 10- We are in the double digits now, and I keep telling myself that we have to get to the big milestone of Day 29 (still in the double digits), so it is not far away. Today was a pretty good day- still a tough day with our steroids. We had to make a stop at the clinic today to get our PICC line flushed, and to check in about some of the diarrhea she has been having over the past day. She is still taking in a good bit of fluids, and is not feverish, so everything appears okay for now. Her PICC line was still giving us some trouble, so they were able to put something in it called TPA (for you medical folks, that will mean something...for me, it is the abbreviation for Tampa airport :) Seriously though, I do understand that it helped to clear anything that would have been blocking her line. We have another clinic appointment on Friday, and one on Monday. One of the doctors we talked to yesterday said that if all is looking well that Taylor may be able to go back to Tallahassee this weekend. Realistically though, we have either been at the clinic or at the hospital every day since we checked out....so it does not look like a feasible option just yet. That is okay though. I am okay with being a few minutes from the hospital. 2 hours away seems like too far at the moment, but maybe a week from now I will feel different...

Taylor has made it clear that she does not like taking her medicine. She is usually pretty angry with her Daddy and me about it. She says it is spicy, and that we are being mean to her. She kicks, punches, and scratches...and her Daddy and I have some marks to prove it...but we still make her take it, and explain that it is helping her cancer germs go away. I've explained to her that there are other people she knows that have had to take cancer germ medicine to get better- like her Great Grandpa, Mr. Saxon next door, her friend Carson, etc. She ends up taking it, but it is not a pleasant experience.

While we were at clinic today, they weighed our little eating machine. She has gained 6 pounds since last week. I am happy to see that she is keeping weight on, and her steroids definitely keep her going. She started the day with 3 bowls of cheese grits...my kind of girl. Daddy was out getting some dinner, and Taylor and I have been watching the 'Sound of Music.' She has really taken a liking to this movie- especially all of the music. Well, Daddy just got back with some dinner, so we'll be signing off for a bit. Take care!

January 31, 2007

We received very good news today. The doctors called us with results from Taylor's biopsy on Monday, and her leukemia counts are less than 4%. That is a goal that is set for the induction period, and for her to reach it by this point in her treatment means that her body is responding well to the treatments to date. Hearing that news made everything over the past 2 weeks...the frustration, everything disappear. Her course of treatment will not change over the induction period, as the standard protocol will still require chemotherapy and additional drug treatments, and she will continue treatments for the next 2 - 3 years. But, we know her body is responding, and with counts less than 4%, the doctors are classifying her as RER (Rapid Early Remission). She is fighting so hard, whether she recognizes it or not.

I've always known she has a strong spirit (That is at least what I told myself when she would throw a public temper tantrum..."she is just a strong-willed child" I would tell myself...and any others observing). Now I know that God had a purpose for that strong will.

Guess what we are watching as I type this? Yes, the Sound of Music. And Taylor's favorite song is the 'So Long, Farewell' song (just like Miss Martha's from her journal update). She has fallen asleep now though. It does seem kind of backwards, but I understand why...her leukemia counts are going down, but I can see the treatments taking quite a toll on her energy. I have to keep reminding myself that her energy levels will go down as the chemo progresses. If these treatments get her better though, that is all that is important.

On a funny note- I know that a good bit of you can imagine how all of this 'Gator' stuff can be overwhelming for Taylor's Daddy. He has probably seen enough orange and blue to last a lifetime, although he has admitted that the Gator doctors and nurses helping her are okay in his book. We take Taylor for drives every day, and we have gone by the stadium as well. So now she recognizes it every time we go by, and says 'That's where the Gators play football.' She knows it is not Doak Campbell or Death Valley, but she likes seeing all of the football stuff around town.

Because her diet has been quite the topic, I will let you know that she finished off a bowl of grits, a bowl of Pistachios, a grilled cheese sandwich, chips and a bowl of spaghetti noodles today. She asked her Daddy to go to the store and get her some pickle spears and some 'Tina' noodles. For those of you from Tallahassee, the 'Tina' noodles she is referring to are from 'Riccardos.' Daddy has headed to Publix, and then Mommy will try her best to make up some Tina noodles for Miss Taylor. I am trying to be thankful for her appetite, as I know it will provide energy for her...

Well, love to all, and I did want to thank everyone again for everything. Taylor has her next clinic visit this Friday, so we will let you know how that goes.

A note for the firefighters out there...someone from my team at work sent me an e-mail that really struck me, and I wanted to share an excerpt of it with you. He wrote the following: "You have every firefighter within a million miles on your side. Remember, these guys go into burning buildings, wrecked cars, they risk everything to save people they don't know (I seem to recall you're married to one) So just think of what they'll do for someone they know and love."

Take care, and we will post additional updates soon.

February 2, 2007

We had intended to update the site yesterday, but were not able to. So, our update is coming on late Friday evening....It has been a pretty long day, but we are thankful that we were still in Gainesville and close to the hospital, as Taylor was re-admitted this afternoon. We had clinic this morning, which was intended to be a standard visit where she would have blood drawn to review her current blood counts. Additionally, she needed a dressing change for her PICC line. When we arrived, her temperature was fine, but as the visit progressed, I could feel her getting warmer. We were also having issues with her PICC line not being cooperative (i.e., they could not draw blood from it). While we were there, the nurses continued to monitor her temperature, which eventually climbed to 100 degrees. While it did not break 100, the doctor was concerned enough to admit her, and said that he would prefer to be conservative, especially during the induction period. So, here we are, but again...thankful that it was a 2-minute drive as opposed to a 2-hour drive. I know that at some point during her battle with this that there will be those times when we will be making a drive from Tallahassee to Shands for an elevated fever; however, I was happy today was not one of those times.

She has been a strong little girl today, and even though

9

she was very upset about having to get another couple of 'pokes' (a new IV in her hand until her PICC line is fixed, and needle sticks in her arm for lab draws), she is doing okay. The doctors are trying to identify if she has any sort of infection that we need to fight, but are just proactively giving her IV antibiotics until the culture results come back. We were due to have another clinic visit on Monday for additional chemotherapy treatment, and I am hopeful that we will be out of the hospital prior to then and can still make that appointment. But if we are not, that is okay- they can still give her the treatment here.

With regard to her PICC line, somehow it has moved (potentially during her dressing change today), and they will need to do a PICC line exchange tomorrow. While I was hopeful that she would be asleep for that procedure, she will not be. They said they would give her something to 'calm her down,' and I explained to the nurse that they better give her a lot of something to 'calm her down.' I just worry that she has been through so much, and I would have preferred that she could be asleep through as much of this as possible, and just think it is all a bad dream.

Her friend Carson from school is here as well fighting an infection, so we had the chance to catch up in person with his Mom tonight. I hate that either Carson or Taylor have to be back in the hospital, but the doctors have explained to us that it is normal to be back in the hospital during induction, especially with their white cell counts so low.

One highlight of our day was during the drive from the clinic to the hospital. Robbie and I had a glimmer of what life was like prior to 2 weeks ago. Out of nowhere, our regular Taylor was with us. She was having conversations about school and Alex and happy things. It wasn't her current day to day attitude that is induced by the steroids. The moment didn't last too long, but it was enough to remind Robbie and I that the medicine is causing so much of her frustration and reactions to us.

We are finishing up Day 13, so almost the half way point of induction...We know she is making progress, and can't think of the hospital admit as a setback. I think it is just a reality of the stage of treatment we are in, and we will get through it.

Before signing off, I do have to thank both Clemson and FSU athletics for their postings and their notes of support for Taylor. Taylor also received a Clemson care package yesterday which she was very excited about- a signed football and basketball as well as clothes, books- just a ton of stuff. And then to balance it out, she wore her head to toe FSU stuff today. She is a good little cheerleader.

Love to everyone, and we will talk to you soon...

February 3, 2007

Thanks for the guestbook postings today. Thankfully, her fever has yet to break 100 degrees, so that is good news. The more challenging part is that she has been a handful and a half since checking back into the hospital. The difference in environment really seems to have an impact on her (understandably), but it is so hard to watch her deal with her frustrations. She was a brave little girl today. The PICC line nurse had to do an exchange on her PICC line so that it would work again. This required doing a procedure in the treatment room. Taylor was awake, but mildly sedated with a drug called Ativan (hoping I spelled that right!). She did great through the procedure, and kept her arm very still. Her PICC line is working again, although we are curious as to when she will have a central line (also called a port) put in her chest. Our understanding is that this will be used as she progresses with her treatment, so definitely a question for the doctors tomorrow. It may be something she has put in during a subsequent procedure when she is asleep...or at least I hope so!

During today's procedure, she was scared and cried a lot, but we had her wrapped up in a papoose and held her tight. When

11

she did talk, all she could talk about was her next snack- a hamburger with cheese (not a cheeseburger mind you, but a hamburger with cheese). Little Taylor continued to eat her way through the hospital today- to the point that was concerning to us though. Her brain is telling her she is hungry, but her belly is definitely full. She basically eats until she gets sick, and then wants to eat some more. Trying to be responsible parents, we are limiting to the extent that we can how much she is intaking. Taking excess food away has caused a lot of her frustration today, so we are hopeful that when she is out of the hospital and has more distractions again (e.g., the park, driving around)she will have things to keep her occupied and keep her mind off of eating non-stop.

Not much more to say about our stay in the hospital at the moment. We are hopeful for her to keep her temperature below 100 degrees, and have a potential discharge from the hospital tomorrow. I told her we could have a Super Bowl party at the hotel. She asked what the colors of the teams were, and I was explaining to her that the Bears are orange and blue. She told me I was wrong, and that those were Gators. We finally met in the middle when I explained to her that she was correct in that their quarterback did used to play for the Gators. She was okay with that answer.

I did want to thank the team of folks who were / are / will be at our house this weekend trying to get it ready for us to come home. I appreciate the coordination of getting the carpets and upholstery cleaned, as well as lysoling / cloroxing the entire house from top to bottom. Please know how much we appreciate it. We are hopeful to be headed home Monday following her chemotherapy treatment. If not Monday, then hopefully later in the week- depending on how she is progressing with maintaining a good temperature.

Take care, and we'll catch up tomorrow (which by the way will be Day 15! So we will be at the half-way point through induction...)

Love, Kim and Rob

February 5, 2007

Taylor was discharged yesterday (Sunday) from the hospital, so we were very happy. While we were there, the doctors explained that between Day 10 and Day 14, they do expect a neutropenic fever. The way that I am understanding the term 'neutropenic' is that she has a highly susceptible immune system (i.e., extremely low white cell count).

So, between Day 10 and 14, the doctors expect these patients to hit their low. Thankfully, her fever did not go over 100 degrees, but more than anything, we needed to get her out of the hospital environment (assuming medically she was okay to go). Her mood swings and outbursts increased while back in the hospital, and unfortunately, she was just hateful to anybody who came to visit. We know that she doesn't truly mean the hateful things she says, but it is hard to remember that consistently (and especially for visitors who aren't inundated with it on a day to day basis- so we apologize).

As I write this, we are having a battle (at 5:30 a.m.) with Taylor over her eating habits. It is really scary how she is addicted to food right now. There is such a balance that we have to walk. You can't deprive her, and we want her to keep weight on, but you can't just let her have everything she wants. If she had her way, she would eat all day long...but it is literally making her sick. So, it is a screaming match all day long because we won't let her eat everything.

We have clinic this morning, during which Taylor will receive some additional chemotherapy. We are also hopeful that her blood counts will come back with good numbers. There is a summary number that the doctors use call an 'ANC' count that factors in her white blood cell count and neutrophils in her body. The doctors want to see it over 500 before she goes back to Tallahassee. During the past few days (what we hope was her lowest), her counts went as low as 52 on

Saturday. We thought they might go all the way to 0, but by Sunday, her ANC had climbed to 260. This was a very positive thing.

Well I need to go, and get the day started...we'll send an update after clinic, and hopefully have a better idea of when we head home...Take care!

February 5, 2007

Day 16 of treatment, and Taylor's ANC was up to 414 today! We found this out during our clinic visit today, and were happy that it is continuing to climb. She also had additional chemotherapy treatment during her visit today, and then was able to come back to the hotel. She is happier being out of the hospital and back to the hotel, and we are hopeful that at her next clinic visit on Thursday that her ANC will be at least 500. If it is, the doctors will most likely let her go home to Tallahassee. We will need to come back next week for additional chemotherapy and a consult with the pediatric surgeon (regarding her central line that will be put in her chest near the end of induction), but I won't mind the commute if she can just get home even for a few days. Her new PICC line is better, and not giving us as much trouble, but it will be good for her to get the central line in as that will be what she has in place for subsequent chemotherapy treatments.

Still fighting the food battle, but we had success today with a new game that Grandma came up with. Grandma disinfected 5 nickels (with lots of Purell), and put them in a special red purse for Taylor. Taylor is allowed to 'buy' 5 snacks per day (Don't worry- she isn't having to buy breakfast, lunch, or dinner, which by the way are pretty big!). These are just for all of her extra snacks during the day. She thought it was a fun game, and actually ate better portions overall today...and didn't make herself sick, which was good. Grandma and Grandpa then spent this evening putting together Ziploc bags of portioned snacks so that Taylor has a 'snack box' that she can buy from each time. Even if the fun of this only lasts for a couple of days, it's at least a couple of days. As she gets past induction, the frequency of the steroid dosages will decrease. Right now she takes them every day, twice per day....I believe that in subsequent phases of her therapy, she will only need to take them 5 days per month. That means that the side effects of the constant appetite and mood swings should start to decrease after Day 29. (We are hoping that to be true!!!)

I wanted to thank Alana, Joy, and Lori for their coordination of two 'Relay for Life' teams for the Godby High School event in April. What a wonderful event, and a great way to support all of those that are battling and beating cancer. The Accenture team is also walking for Niki McDowell, the son of one of my coworkers. Niki has been making great strides in his treatment, and has amazed everyone. Since the time that all of this has started with Taylor, I have not had the opportunity to tell Jay (Niki's dad) that he and his wife have been role models in how to handle this whole experience. They are a model of optimism with their experience with Niki, and I can only hope to continue to be that positive. I'm sure that our attitudes will have such an impact on Taylor's perception of this and how she approaches it.

In anticipation of Taylor coming home on Thursday, Rob has made a day trip up to Tallahassee to take some stuff home and to get things settled for Taylor. Alex has been spending time with both families over the past 2 weeks, which we are very appreciative of....and we have had the chance to see her each weekend. It is hard for the 4 of us to be apart though, and are looking forward to having all of us back in one place very soon.

Well, love to all, and I am going to sleep now. Miss Taylor is sleeping now, but will be up early with a grumbling tummy....Take care, and hope to see everyone very soon.

February 7, 2007

I fell asleep last night before getting a chance to update the journal....just really tired!

Taylor had an amazing day yesterday. She had very few outbursts, and overall was very happy and more sociable. Her nickel game continued to work, and we ate a little more reasonably...Grandpa had stayed with us yesterday while Rob was gone, and she was just talking up a storm with him. He made her spaghetti for dinner, and he was her hero. She still had her moments, especially when it was time to take medicine, but the medicine still went down, so I can't ask for more than that. She also did a good job of taking some walks yesterday. We are really trying to keep an eye on her legs and any pain she complains of. One of the side effects of the chemotherapy is weakening of her leg muscles and neuropathy (which would adversely impact her walking), so we want to keep an eye on it and get any sort of physical therapy going if needed. The only thing we've noticed in the past couple of days is that she is having trouble lifting her legs high enough to put on pants when she is getting dressed. I'll mention it to the doctor tomorrow, but she is still walking (and galloping too!)

Another reason yesterday was amazing was that Taylor and I spent a lot of time talking. Grandpa was working at the hotel, and Taylor and I went to the park to play. We ended up opening up the back door of the van, and setting up a picnic in the back of the van. When we were done eating, she laid down on my lap for about an hour and let me stroke her hair, and she asked me to talk to her about various things..."Tell me about when I was a baby mommy and I drank bottles...Tell me about when Alex was born...Tell me about you and Daddy getting married..." I just talked and talked to her, and she laid there so still and relaxed. As I was talking to her, I was looking around at the park, breathing deep, and couldn't remember the last time I had slowed down and taken time to appreciate the time together the past few weeks has resulted in. In light of everything else going on, I do appreciate the fact that I had time to focus on something like having that conversation with my daughter without any consideration of rushing off to the next activity or appointment- this is the only thing on my plate right now.

Someone sent us a book recently called 'When God and Cancer Meet.' I have started reading the book, and it includes various stories about people impacted by cancer (both patients and the people close to them). The author, a cancer survivor herself, has put together a great group of stories that show how God touched each of the people during their experience with cancer. In the author's words 'Sometimes God took the cancer out of them, and sometimes he took them out of the cancer...but always, he touched them with his divine love and met their deepest needs.' This has been a good book to start reading during our experience, and to keep in mind there is a bigger plan for all of this, one that we still may not fully understand. An excerpt I read yesterday really stuck out to me. It said 'Give yourself time to absorb all that has been thrown at you, and give God time to make something new and good from the shattered pieces.' Not sure yet what this will all be, but I do know that I am consciously going to slow down more than I have in the past, and truly appreciate and be thankful for all of the blessings in my life. I only thought I was appreciative before. Now I think additional perspective has been thrown on top of that.

We have a clinic appointment tomorrow, so hopefully her ANC is above 500...which will be the go ahead to head home to Tallahassee for the weekend. During her appointment, we will also have the chance to meet with Dr. Hunger, the Chief of the Pediatric Hematology / Oncology department here at Shands. So I will let everyone know if he sheds light on any other progress or key milestones we are shooting for...Right now, we are focused on February 19th...the end of induction.

Alrighty- it is time to watch the Wiggles for a little bit with Taylor. I think these are the same songs from yesterday, but that's okay. Talk to you soon, and hopeful to be writing this from Tallahassee as of tomorrow!

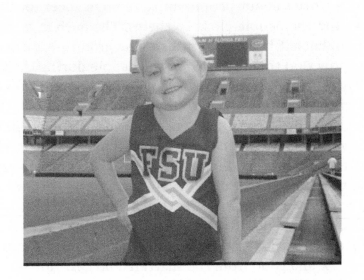

HOMEWARD BOUND

February 8, 2007

We are at home in Tallahassee...what a wonderful thing! Hopefully the start of getting back some normalcy for Taylor.

Taylor was welcomed home to a 'princess themed mural' that Cinderella painted in her room while she was gone. Thank you to all of Cinderella's helpers who did the painting over the past week. She just loved it. She came up the stairs, looked into her room, and said "What? Mommy look at my room! Cinderella made it green and pink, and there is a castle, and a glass slipper..." We asked her if she liked it, and she said yes....and then she asked "Did Cinderella paint your room too?"

We had a clinic appointment in Gainesville this morning, during which we were able to meet with Dr. Hunger, one of Taylor's doctors. He did let us know that her ANC was at 390, but he felt that this was acceptable for this point in her treatment, and was comfortable with her going home. Knowing that he knows a heck a lot more about this stuff than me, I figured that if he wasn't nervous about the ANC not being higher, I wouldn't be overly concerned. While he had previously mentioned that he would prefer that the ANC be over 500 before she went home, he also mentioned that we were coming back in just a couple of days for additional treatments...so I'm sure that factored into the ability for us to come home for the weekend today. We will head back to Gainesville next week for additional chemotherapy and for Taylor to get her PICC line removed. Dr. Hunger said that it appears to be giving her unnecessary trouble, and that it would be better to get her port in sooner than later. With that in mind, she will also have a follow-up lumbar puncture (LP) and bone marrow biopsy late next week. During that procedure, her port will be put in. We will understand more after the consult next week with the pediatric surgeon, but my understanding is that the port runs less of a chance for infection than the PICC line, and will continue to be used for chemotherapy treatments going forward.

While it is great to be home, I think it is a little overwhelming for Taylor too. We do have to continue to be sensitive to the fact that she is still in the induction period, with an extremely low white blood cell count, and very susceptible to infection. This means that we will pretty much continue to be in seclusion from visitors for at least another week. We did take a walk outside today, and said hello to our friends in the neighborhood, but she is a little withdrawn right now. I think she is feeling a lot of things- tired, still scared, and not understanding why she has been gone from her home and friends for 3 weeks....and why she can't go inside anybody else's house right now. This would be a lot for anyone to take on, let alone a 3-year-old...

Well, Taylor is taking a nap at the moment, but I will eventually need to wake her up to take her medicine before she goes to bed for the night...so take care, and we'll keep everyone posted!

February 10, 2007

This is my first attempt at updating the journal so please bear with me. I was back at the Fire Station today after a three week stay in Hogtown, Kim and Taylor went to the park and had a picnic lunch. Taylor is very happy to be back in Tallahassee in her own bed with her own toys. Grandma is meeting Aunt Kathy tomorrow to pick up Alex who has been in Port St Lucie with Gammy for a week. Taylor is so excited to see her.

We go back to clinic on Tuesday for more chemotherapy and to have our pic line removed, just a day trip.

Kim and Taylor are sleeping, Kim needs her rest she is running a 5K tomorrow. Taylor and I are going to watch and cheer her on. Well I better go it's getting late, Kim will update more tomorrow.

February 10, 2007

I think Robbie did a fine job with his update yesterday....and I did want to get out an update to everyone that Taylor is continuing to do better at home. She was so excited to see Alex today. Alex ran up to her and gave her 2 big hugs....and then tried to take Taylor's turkey and cheese sandwich. I probably don't have to tell you how that went over. Taylor made it pretty clear that 'We don't share food Alex.' Our biggest battles at the moment continue to be taking medicine (it gets taken, but it is a good 20-minute struggle), and some challenges controlling potty accidents (trying to say that nicely). I've tried to explain to Taylor that the medicine can make our bodies have to go potty a lot more, and that wearing training pants may be a good idea, but she is very frustrated by that part. She tells me that she is not a baby. We're just trying to help her understand that it is temporary.

I was very appreciative that Robbie and Taylor came out to the race today. With everything going on, I felt slightly selfish about still doing the race today, but I wanted to follow through on it, and I have to remember that it will be important to keep going with some of the things that Robbie and I used to do...I am new to this whole running thing, and along with 3 good friends (Julie, Lori, and Angie), we have been supporting each other in getting ready for this 5-K....although, thanks to a little divine intervention today, I may be asking those 3 ladies to start training for the Leukemia and Lymphoma Society marathon in San Diego (don't worry ladies, we'll shoot for next year's running of it...we do need a little time to train). While at the race today, I noticed that there were several people with t-shirts on that said something about the Leukemia and Lymphoma Society. I got talking to one gentleman about it, and he explained that he was training for a marathon in San Diego and was raising money for cancer research. I explained to him that Taylor had just been diagnosed in January, and he said that he would love to chat when we met up at the finish line. When I got there, I had the opportunity to meet some of the other folks who are training for the marathon, and chat a little more about Taylor. It turns out that the coach knew a mutual friend (the coordinator of Taylor's princess room mural!), and said that they had been praying for Taylor. It makes me remember what a small world it is, and reminds me of how divine intervention plays a role in our lives. She asked if Rob and I would be interested in attending an upcoming breakfast and speaking to the group to remind / help inspire the reason for their marathon. I told her that we would be more than happy to do that, as I am so appreciative that there are folks out there that are focused on this cause.

Well, Miss Taylor is sleeping now, so I will probably try to get some sleep myself soon. We are finishing up Day 21 of induction, and Day 29 gets closer each day...I am hopeful that once we get past induction that we can have visitors to the house. While she can play outside, we are still trying to be very careful about visitors at the house for the near future. When we do start having visitors again, I will ask you to leave your shoes at the door :), and to wear a mask if you have come within 100 feet of someone with a cold that day (just kidding about the 100 feet, but don't be offended if there are masks out). We are just taking guidance from the doctors and nurses from Shands, and trying to do everything in our power to keep her germ free while she is so immune suppressed. Have a good evening, and thank you again for your postings...your prayers are working...

Love, Kim, Rob, Taylor and Alex

February 11, 2007

Day 22 is coming to a close- only 1 week left of induction. There are times when it feels like the days are dragging, but then I see we are on Day 22 already, and it feels like it is flying too. I am happy to say that we made huge strides taking our medicine tonight. While she still put up a little bit of a fight verbally, there was no crying. That is the first time that has ever happened...and I think from start to finish, it took her less than 5 minutes to take all of her various medicines. Rob and I often wonder if she will eventually just accept that the medicine has to be taken, and that we are not going to throw it away (even though she asks us each time...'Mommy and Daddy, please just throw that spicy medicine away'). Aunt Debbie was here tonight while she took her medicine, and promised Taylor that we will have a 'No more yucky medicine party' when all of the yucky medicine is done. Taylor is excited about planning that.

She had a nice day with Daddy today. Mommy, Grandma and Alex were out running some errands, so Daddy and Taylor had some nice quality time together. I was very happy that she went on a walk in the stroller today, and went around the block 5 times with her Daddy.

As nice as it was to have Alex home this weekend, it was also a little more challenging than I think I was willing to admit. Taylor was very loving at times to Alex and protective as well (i.e., she didn't want anyone else talking to Alex except her); however, there were times when Taylor would have outbursts during which Alex would get very upset and scared. Additionally, when Taylor woke up at night screaming, Alex heard her and woke up too... so then we then had 2 little ones awake and not wanting to go back to sleep. With that in mind, and recognizing that we only have 1 week left of induction (and daily steroids), I thought it was best to ask my Mom and Dad to keep Alex for the week until we get closer to the end of induction. It is hard for me to admit that I don't think I will have the energy this week for both of them for those times that I will be here by myself....but induction will be done at the end of this week, and the doctors have explained that the side effects from the steroids will wear off after the end of induction. I also don't want Taylor's illness to overshadow the need for Alex to have personal attention. Between Rob's family and my family, Alex has received that attention and love by staying with both families over the past few weeks. As much as we miss her, I think it would hurt worse to see her not get the attention she needs and deserves...I think we will be in a better place next week as we (hopefully) move into the next phase of Taylor's treatment called 'Consolidation.' I have to read up on it, but I will let everyone know exactly what that means. I heard another mom compare it to a pregnancy's three trimesters. With Leukemia (ALL) treatment, you go through three phases: Induction, Consolidation, and Maintenance. Thankfully, induction is not scheduled to be 3 months! The specific roadmap and drug treatments for Taylor's 'Consolidation' phase will be determined as we wrap up induction and have specifics about her leukemia cell counts, blood counts, and results of genetic studies.

She is such a brave little girl, and it saddens her daddy and me to watch her little body go through this. The medicine has taken its toll already. Her cheeks are very puffy, her belly is pooched out from weight gain and water retention, her body is bruised in areas where the skin is stretching, it is hard sometimes for her to control her moods, and her hair is beginning to thin out. What's odd about her hair is that we keep preparing ourselves for it to fall out, and it hasn't yet. While it looks thinner, I'm not finding strands anywhere yet- not on the pillows or in her brush. While that's not a bad thing, I do wonder where it is going then. While it will be hard for us to see her with no hair (because I think it reinforces to us that she is sick), I do wonder if she will be upset about it. Other moms I've talked to said that their daughters barely care about it, and don't even care to wear hats sometimes. I only wish that as adults we could all be that self-confident and not even factor in others' thoughts and stares.

Well, she is sleeping peacefully right now, so I will probably opt for an early bedtime myself. Love to everyone, and take care.

February 12, 2007

Day 23 is wrapping up, and we just got Taylor settled to bed. We have clinic in Gainesville tomorrow, with the intent of coming home tomorrow afternoon. She is okay about going tomorrow, because she thinks of it as the 'turkey and cheese place.' (i.e., they give her a box lunch each time she is there for a treatment, and to date it has always included a turkey and cheese sandwich). We are hopeful that her ANC (blood count calculation) is up tomorrow, and continues to indicate progress. While we are planning to come home tomorrow, we will still pack a suitcase to be prepared...but I hope it stays packed and returns home that way!

She had a pretty good day today. We took a field trip to the fire station to visit Daddy today, and she wore her mask so that the germs would stay away. It was nice to visit the fire station and for her to see the trucks. She always has her Daddy take her to see the trucks when she visits. On the way to pick up lunch today, she told me she missed her friends from school, and that she wanted them to come over and play. I explained that we might have to wait a little longer to have everyone over, but that maybe we could have someone over to play outside. She understood that we couldn't have anybody inside yet, but she asked if I would call Jenna's mommy to see if she could play outside. Jenna came over this afternoon, but Taylor wasn't feeling the best at that time. She was in a pretty bad mood actually. I explained that she has her good moments, but then can quickly switch to bad moods....but that hopefully after induction wraps up, we will see a decrease in the mood swings. Jenna and her mommy were very understanding, and as much as I wish they could have played today, it may have just been too soon. I just know that Taylor misses her friends and school...and I wish we could give her that right now.

More strands of hair fell out today. I am starting to notice that it is thinner. Like I was saying in yesterday's update, it is so hard to watch her little body go through this. We do have some things to talk to the doctor about tomorrow- as she is having some blood in her stool when she goes potty, and the site where she had her bone marrow biopsy is continuing to 'weep.' That is the term that Robbie used, so it must be a technical term :), but essentially, it continues to leak clear fluid. It is not red or infected, (which is what the doctors asked when we called Shands about it), but it is constantly leaking fluid. It is almost as if her body is holding so much fluid, and the skin is stretching so much, that the water has no place else to go but to leak out of this site. Hopefully they will be able to give us some more insight tomorrow about that. She is having some pain when trying to get comfortable sitting, and we worked on our deep breathing exercises today (flash back to childbirth classes). She is a good little breather though, and breathes really good when she is feeling pain. She will be ready for Lamaze when she needs to be.

Love to all, and we will post an update from clinic as soon as we have a chance.

February 13, 2007

Great news today! We had our clinic visit, and her ANC was up to 1800! That is up from 390 during her visit last Thursday. Her white blood cell count is up to 5.0 from 1.3 (normal range starts at 10, so we are getting there!), and her platelets were up as well. All signs are currently indicating that she is responding well to treatment. We still have a long road ahead of us, but it is encouraging to have these points along the way.

She did very well at clinic, and was really talkative with all of the nurses. She brought them some of her Valentine's cupcakes, and made sure that they ate them 'all gone.' (her words...) Overall, she seemed to feel pretty comfortable at clinic today which was nice. The nurses and doctors at Shands are really amazing. They do all that they can to make sure the kids are comfortable. They have little DVD screens set up at each treatment station, so that the kids can play PlayStation or watch a movie. To date, Taylor has watched 'Dora's Halloween' every time.

It was nice to come home with our suitcase still packed! We will be back down in Gainesville later this week for some additional procedures, but planning to come back the same day.

Well, Taylor is resting, but sleeping pretty light right now, so I will sign off for the night. We'll let you know how the little princess is doing tomorrow. We're on to Day 25 tomorrow!

February 14, 2007

I wanted to focus tonight's journal update with a request for everyone to keep a special family in your prayers. McKenzie, a little girl that Taylor met at Shands passed away this weekend. We found out today, and it was a pretty impactful moment. Our thoughts and prayers are with McKenzie's family, and we are so thankful that we were able to spend the time that we did with McKenzie and her family. Her parents are wonderful, strong people, and sought us out at the hospital when they heard we were from Tallahassee. McKenzie's mom spent time stopping by our room to check in and to give us pointers about how to adjust and cope with the diagnosis. As her obituary read today, Mckenzie "was granted her angel wings Feb. 11, 2007, following a two-year battle with cancer." I know she is in a better place, and a place where there is no more pain or cancer, but I can only imagine the sadness her family must be feeling right now. Please keep them in your prayers, and know that heaven has yet another guardian angel.

February 15, 2007

Day 26 is about wrapped up, and we are headed to Gainesville early in the morning for Taylor's next bone marrow biopsy, a lumbar puncture, and for the pediatric surgeon to put her port in her chest. It sounds like a busy day, but I believe all of the procedures should not take more than a couple of hours to complete. She had an okay day, but then we've had a great evening. She took her medicine better than she ever has, and then she and I were talking and had one of those "park moments" again (for those of you who read my previous journal entries, you may remember the day at the park I described where Taylor and I had great conversation). She had just gotten dressed for bed, and her Daddy had run to the store for some Gatorade...and she wanted to tell me all about school and the playground there. She went into all sorts of details about the toys at school, her teachers, and all of her friends there, and how she wants her friends and teachers from school to come to her house and play when she is feeling better. She said that she would like to have them all come to her house and then go out to eat for spaghetti noodles (interesting get together she is coming up with, but I loved listening to her talk about it). She would prefer not to have any sauce on her spaghetti because it might hurt her lips, but meatballs sound really yummy. When we first started talking, my mind was racing about "all of the things I needed to get done tonight" (i.e., rinse out the syringes from her medicine she just took, pack our things for tomorrow's trip, re-clorox the house from top to bottom....), but then I remembered that the conversation was much more important than any of that, and that all of those things can be done when she falls asleep shortly. I really treasure the conversations we've been having this past month.

She is really an amazing kid, and I give her a lot of credit for how she is handling all of the 'new knowledge' she has acquired this past month. She throws out medical terms and names of her medicines from time to time, and she is coming around to her visits she needs to make to Gainesville. One of the best pieces of advice that the nurses gave us at Shands was to never lie to her about her treatments or medicines (i.e., Don't say that the shot won't hurt....or that the medicine doesn't taste bad). Be honest with her. Tell her the medicine tastes bad, but she does have to take it to get better. I think we would all agree that honesty is the best policy, but as a parent, I'm sure that I have fibbed a billion times when I thought it would protect my child. This experience has taught me that when it comes to the various procedures and medicines, etc. that Taylor has to go through- there is no sugar coating it. We have to be honest with her. For example, I have been dreading the fact that she cannot have anything to eat after midnight tonight (in preparation for her procedures tomorrow). With her recent appetite, you can imagine how much that was stressing us out. However, I sat down with her tonight and explained that the doctors need her belly to be empty tomorrow when they see her or they won't be able to do all of their check-ups and tests. I promised her that when we are done visiting the doctors that we can go eat whatever she wants. She said 'That's okay Mommy, I just won't eat in the morning.' Now, let's just hope that it goes that smoothly when we wake up!

Well, I know this has been a long update, so I will sign off for now. Tomorrow will bring us more news of the status of progression in her treatment, and the intent is to have enough progression to begin moving into the 'Consolidation' phase of treatment. We will let you know how it goes....Love to all, and thank you for the continued prayers, cards, treats for Taylor- all of it has kept all of our spirits high.

February 16, 2007

Good news...we are in transit back from Gainesville. Rob has figured out how to use his phone as a modem, so we can be extra efficient and get computer stuff done in the car too (don't worry- the passenger, not the driver). Taylor had her procedures done today, and we expect the results from her LP and her bone marrow biopsy on Monday. The doctors were very hopeful, and even mentioned that when they did the bone marrow biopsy today that the marrow was flowing out. This is a stark contrast to a few weeks ago where the doctor said it was hard to get any bone marrow out of her because all of the leukemia cells were crowding the marrow out. So even though we don't have final results, we are hopeful that things are continuing to progress.

She also had her central line put in today, and her PICC line taken out. While she may be a little sore for a couple of days, having the central line should be a good thing going forward. It will allow her to take regular baths, swim this summer...overall, it will be much more flexible than the PICC line.

She is in a good mood now, but she was pretty hungry this morning (with not being able to eat prior to the procedures). Even though we had talked about it last night, I think she was pretty convinced that her daddy and I were trying to starve her. She told us that we were being mean to her and wouldn't feed her, and that she won't be our friends. When all was done, we went through Wendy's, and now I think we are on her good list again. Well, we will sign off for now, as we are almost back to Tallahassee and have to run into Publix. We are running low on turkey and bread- and we know that Miss Taylor will want a turkey and cheese sandwich at some point today.

Take care, and we'll post more later...

Love, Kim and Rob

February 17, 2007

Taylor and mommy just got home from running a couple of errands, including a new haircut. Miss Mary at Athena Salon gave Taylor a very pretty, short haircut today. When we got to the salon, we looked through magazines and picked a pretty haircut just like the movie stars. She landed on a picture of Alyssa Milano with a short haircut (which I think Taylor wears beautifully). Miss Mary asked her if she wanted any gel in it to make it spiky and fun, but Taylor passed on that for now. We'll post a picture of her new haircut when she's ready. Lately (and I understand), she hasn't been excited about pictures. She told me 'I'm sick and I don't want my picture taken...' so we have respected her wishes...If she doesn't want any pictures for the foreseeable future, that is fine too.

I did want to let everyone know about a wonderful event coming up that is sponsored by the Tallahassee Professional Firefighters Union (to visit their website, go to http:// www.iafflocal2339.org/). The event is a benefit ball for 'Burn Camp' and for Taylor. Burn Camp is an annual event supported by the Tallahassee Firefighters and it is held at Cape San Blas. It is a summer camp for kids ages 6-18 that are burn survivors. We are appreciative that the firefighters offered to include Taylor as part of this benefit, and wanted to make people aware of the date and additional information about it. From the union website, you will find links to the benefit ball (scheduled for April 21st at 8 p.m. at the American Legion Hall). There will be some great performances. There will be more information about tickets as the date gets closer, but mark your calendars now! The Tallahassee Firefighters support great causes, and we can't thank them enough for how much they have supported us. I also wanted to thank them for including information about Taylor on their website, and a link to her web page. It has helped to direct people to the website for her updates...

Today has been a great day so far. Alex is coming home, and Taylor is excited about that. Additionally, tonight will be her last dose of steroids for a while. While she will continue on other various medications, the steroids can stop for now.

I think this is also good timing with Alex coming home. It should help the mood swings which will hopefully minimize any outbursts for now....and her appetite may take a break for a bit too. She is trying to recognize when she is full, but like we've explained to her....her brain keeps telling her hungry, even when her belly can't fit any more!

This weekend will wrap up her induction period, and we are scheduled for our next clinic visit on Thursday. So assuming that all goes well this week, we will be moving to the next phase of her treatment shortly.

Well, I hope that everyone is having a nice weekend. We'll look forward to seeing

everyone soon. Taylor is especially excited to meet her friend Madison's new baby brother that was just born the other day. She is excited that Madison is a big sister too! Congratulations to the Bellamy family, and we hope to see you soon.

Love, Kim, Rob, Taylor and Alex

February 18, 2007

Sunday night, and the end of the induction period....today was the first day we didn't have to give Taylor a dose of steroids. While it will take a few days for the effects to wear off, it was a happy day. We were reading through another little one's website, and I think they describe it much more realistically than we have...the fact that you are always on eggshells, not knowing what is going to set her off...having to force her not to eat. We know it's not her fault, but it is such a trying time. The doctors explained to us that there will be another period of time coming up called "delayed intensification" where Taylor will be on another 29-day regimen of the same induction period treatment. The intent is to have another round of intensive treatment to make sure that the cancer germs stay gone. Through years of research and trial and error, this is something that has proven to help with the cure rate, so that is what we will do. While I am not looking forward to the side effects from delayed intensification, if it is best for Taylor- that is of course what we will do.

She was okay smiling for the camera today for a picture of her new haircut, but she told me that it hurt for her to smile right now. While she doesn't look like the same Taylor that she did a month ago, we know it is, and I'm sure we will see her go through many more changes before this is all over.

Grandma kept an eye on the girls for us tonight while Rob and I got out for dinner. It was good to talk and take stock of everything and the perspective that this experience has taught us to date. I'm sure there is so much more to come. It is hard sometimes to see normal life going on around you. I wish every day that I could "stress" again about trying to get Taylor from school and to gymnastics on time....or figure out how to get her to get matching clothes on. Wow- this is definitely a new perspective.

Mom, Aunt Debbie, and Taylor played at home today while Alex and I went to Publix. It was the first time I had been to our Publix in over a month. It was an awesome trip. I soaked in every aisle. I will never take trips to the store for granted again....

We can't thank everyone enough for your continued following of Taylor's progress. For those that post regular updates, and for those that may log in to the website on a regular basis to read journal updates- we appreciate it. It really keeps us going. Take care, and we'll post more tomorrow....love, Rob, Kim, Taylor and Alex

February 19, 2007

Today was a beautiful day outside, and I was happy that Taylor made the suggestion to have a picnic at the park. While we try to encourage it, she hasn't wanted to spend a ton of time outside lately, so every time she suggests it, we are quick to agree. We had a picnic in the tailgate of Daddy's truck, and then it was time to come home and rest. Today was a day of lots of puzzles, and learning how to share toys again with Alex. One interesting thing about the girls being apart for a month is that neither of them have had to share in a month either....they will get over that soon enough! Many thanks to Miss Elissa for the yummy spaghetti dinner tonight. Taylor loved it, and I will have to follow up for the recipe!

The effects of the steroids are still with us, although we are noticing some decrease in the number of outbursts during the day. The appetite is definitely still there, and so difficult to control, but I also realize that there will be times during her treatment where she won't want to eat at all. I'm sure that we will be even more worried about that. My heart just broke this morning when she woke up crying about leg pain in both legs. She wanted me to massage her legs to help it go away. Eventually, the pain must have subsided, and she was able to walk decently today, so hopefully she is doing okay.

We are appreciative that folks are already excited about the upcoming benefit event on April 21st sponsored by the Tallahassee Professional Firefighters Union (to visit their website, go to http://www.iafflocal2339.org/). Please check out the link, and your calendars. The event benefits both the annual 'Burn Camp' that the firefighters sponsor as well as our little Taylor...

We have not heard back about the biopsy results from last Friday yet, but hope to soon. We will post some news as soon as we have it. Our next visit to clinic is this Thursday, and one battle we are currently fighting is some skin breakdown that she has on her bottom. The doctors have given us some medicine to apply in hopes that it will resolve itself quickly. Unfortunately, she cannot move onto the next round of chemotherapy until all infections and skin breakdown are resolved...so that is a goal for this week too.

Well, love to all, and hopefully we will have results to post shortly about her bone marrow biopsy.

Love, Kim, Rob, Taylor and Alex

February 21, 2007

We received good news tonight! Around 7:00 pm, one of Taylor's doctors called and let us know that Taylor's bone marrow biopsy results show that she continues to be in remission! This was so reassuring to hear- knowing that her body is continuing to respond to the treatment. There are still a lot of treatments and procedures to come, including 3 biopsy procedures over the next 3 weeks, but it is just part of protocol, so we are ready to do whatever we need to for her. The doctor explained that a detailed report will be available when we are at clinic this week that will provide an exact statistic about her status, but that these initial results show her in a category of having less than 5% leukemia cells left. For example, she could have less than 4% or less than 1%, and the detailed report will help us better understand that.

Today was a good day overall. After some time at home this morning, the family took an outing to drop off a 'big sister' gift to Taylor's friend Madison whose Mommy just had a baby boy. While she understood that it just meant a trip to Madison's front porch (with a promise to play together real soon!), it was a nice outing for her. We followed that with a trip to Chik-Fil-A, and a picnic outside at home with Alex at her Princess picnic table. She and Alex then had a good time blowing bubbles outside. The effect of the steroids seemed to be a little less today, so that was nice. It was interesting- she still wanted us to make a lot of food today, but then she couldn't finish it. That may be the start of a decreasing appetite, so that was good. As I said last night, I'm sure at some point that I will wish she is eating more, so I know this will continue to be a tough balance.

She carried around a new friend named 'Germy' today. Germy is a present that one of our friends (Miss Kathryn) sent along to Taylor. Germy helped Miss Kathryn out at one point, and is now helping Taylor out too. I explained to her that Germy is helping take all of the cancer germs away, and that he will keep them for Taylor. She brought him to the fire station today for a visit. She left him in the car when we got home tonight, and she asked me to go out and get him so that he could come back inside. He is back on the table now watching over her and waiting to catch some more of those germs for her. With results like we heard today, he must be doing his job!

I've talked to various folks over the past couple of days who said that after seeing Taylor's recent picture that it somehow 'makes all of this real.' I know what you mean, and it is okay to be thinking that. I'm not offended when I hear that, and please don't feel bad about talking to us about that. It makes it very real for us too. It's hard to see her little body going through this, and to hear some of her friends with questions about 'Why does Taylor look so different?'

Believe me, when we were initially in the hospital for treatments, I kept on thinking that Taylor doesn't 'look sick,' and 'maybe she won't have all the side effects that we've heard about.' But then, you watch her little body transform from the various medicines. She's gained more than 12 pounds in a 2-week period. That's tough on anyone's body. And with a decreasing appetite, she will probably lose weight too. She now has a variety of clothes to help accommodate various sizes until that stabilizes. Today, she literally pulled out clumps of hair in her hand. At first she thought it was funny, but then she told her Daddy and I that she wanted her long hair back, and then asked 'If I wash my hair, will it grow longer?' That is a tough comment to respond to- because you can't sugarcoat it. You know it's not coming back until it all falls out, and then who knows how long that will take? So we just explained to her that the medicine is going to make it get even shorter, and that eventually all of her hair will fall out. But then after that point, it will grow back, and we will let it grow back really long. I'm not going to rush out and buy wigs just yet though. She may come to terms with it, and not want wigs, etc. And other moms have mentioned to me that their kids explain that the wigs are too itchy, so we will let this whole thing just play out, and we will help her cope with it the way that seems to work best for her. So, after saying all that- I know what you mean when you say that 'this makes it real...' because it does.

Take care, and thank you for your continued prayers. Robbie and I were discussing that there are miracles we are praying for, including her full recovery, but God is also granting us miracles along the way. From the time the diagnosis was ALL (Pre-B), it was a blessing in itself because of her chances for a cure. Her biopsy results along the way have been a miracle, including going into rapid early remission by Day 9 of treatment. We have been really blessed with these miracles to date.

Love to all, and we will talk to you soon...

February 22, 2007

Great news, we moved into consolidation today. Taylor's labs were great and Dr. Hunger moved her up early. Kim is in Gainesville tonight with Taylor and Alex and I will be joining them tomorrow morning. Taylor will have chemo tomorrow morning. Thanks to everyone who has been keeping up with her progress.

Taylor was feeling photogenic yesterday, check out the new photos. Thank you

Rob, Kim, Taylor, Alex

February 23, 2007

As Rob mentioned in the update from yesterday, Taylor has now moved on to the 'Consolidation' phase. We are very excited. To move into 'Consolidation,' her blood counts had to be at a certain level, and the doctors needed to be comfortable with her progress and health....so it is very good news to us that they wanted her to move forward. So far, it has essentially been a shifting of the medicine regimen, and there are the continued visits to clinic and procedures to help monitor her progress. She had chemotherapy treatments both yesterday and today, and her daily medication has changed so that she is taking a new pill called 6-MP (short for Mercaptopurine). My understanding is that this is an oral form of chemotherapy medicine. Since she takes this in pill form, we crush it up each night with applesauce. So Taylor just calls this her 'applesauce medicine.' I cannot even tell you how much easier it has been the past 2 days to give her this medicine! She only has to take it once per day....that is a big change from the multiple medicines twice per day!

We were also so proud of Taylor both yesterday and today with regard to how she handled the nurses accessing and deaccessing her port. For those of you not familiar with what I mean....the port is under her skin, and is accessed using a needle each time it is needed. While that sounds pretty yucky, there is a special numbing cream that is applied to her chest (where the port is) prior to them accessing it. The nurses also sprayed it with 'freezy spray' (again, probably a more technical name, but that is what they told her it was called), and then they stick the needle into the port. She didn't even cry. I think this was for a variety of reasons, including the fact that the nurses were so patient and took the time to explain to her what they were doing and that the cream helped it not to hurt. Additionally, they did some role playing with 'chemo duck' prior to accessing Taylor's port. Taylor carried chemo duck with her everywhere yesterday and today, including into her 'lumbar puncture' (LP) procedure today. Chemo duck came to the recovery room with a band-aid on his back too- just like Taylor. I can't say enough about how the doctors and nurses at Shands go above and beyond to help the kids feel comfortable...even making sure the duck has all the same stuff that Taylor does. The LP today was done in order to give Taylor more chemotherapy directly into her spine. These will continue for the next few weeks during 'Consolidation.'

After our trip to Gainesville, we continued south to Grandma and Grandpa's house. In addition to a change of scenery, there are extra hands to help with the girls for a few days. It will also give us a chance to see Gammy and Aunt Kathy who are traveling over from Port St. Lucie tomorrow. Taylor has been on cloud 9 since we got to Sarasota today. We haven't seen her this happy in a long time. She is smiling, laughing, playing outside....Her daddy heard her laughing over the phone tonight, and said he couldn't remember the last time he heard her laugh this hard. She has been off of the steroids for 5 days now. Her attitude is much happier, her appetite is slowly going back to normal, and she is starting to drop a lot of the water weight which helps her feel more comfortable.

Well, I am off to bed soon. It has been a long day! Thank you for all of your continued prayers, support and postings. We read them every day....

Love, Rob, Kim, Taylor and Alex

February 24, 2007

The days just keep getting better this week. She laughed and smiled so much today...it was just amazing. Miss Taylor started off her day by helping Grandpa make pancakes and straight sausages (link sausages, but she prefers to call them straight sausages). It was her job to be the 'bubble watcher' for the pancakes and tell Grandpa when to flip them. Breakfast was delicious, and then we moved on to going for a walk to see the ducks and turtles in a nearby pond. I was so proud of her because she asked if I could push Alex in the stroller while she pedalled on her little bike. She rode her bike to the pond and back (very good exercise for her legs). She fed the ducks and the turtles some Cheerios, and then it was time to head back home for a bit. She stayed with Grandma to play sidewalk chalk while Alex and I ran to Target for some clothes for Taylor. She has lost so much water weight this week that she is now back down 2 sizes....and it is much warmer in Sarasota than it is in Tallahassee, so we traded in some sweat pants for some shorts and t-shirts today. Additionally, with the sun shining so bright here, it was definitely time to pick up a sun hat for Miss Taylor (with a matching one for Alex of course).

We had a really fun visit today with Gammy and Aunt Kathy. They drove over from Port Saint Lucie and spent the day with us. We went on a picnic to the park, and drove around town. We played at the house, and had a cook-out tonight too. Taylor and Alex even posed for some pictures (to be posted tomorrow though- I'll be headed to bed soon tonight!)

It was a stark contrast to the last visit that Gammy and Kathy had with Taylor a few weeks back when she was in the midst of her induction period. She was in the hospital, and was constantly in some sort of steroid-induced outburst. Before it got dark out tonight, she even took Kathy outside to pick oranges and grapefruits for Uncle Jack. She is in great spirits.

I know that induction was a trying time for Rob and I, but I can also imagine that it was so hard on any visitors who had taken the time to come see us. She did not want anything to do with people who came to see her, and was often very nasty; however, we know that it wasn't our little girl....she is coming back to us now!

She seems to be doing well with her new medicine. She lost a good bit of hair today, but I don't know whether to attribute that to the new medicine or just to the fact that it was going to come out anyway. One challenge we ran into yesterday at the hospital was that several people kept calling her a 'boy' instead of a 'girl' (For example, a nurse she hadn't met before asked 'How is he doing today?') I can't fault them, as I made this mistake myself in the hospital...however, I will remember to dress her in pink and/or in girly looking stuff as much as possible. It just so happened that she had on navy blue pants yesterday and a shirt that said 'My dad's a rock star...' so it is understandable that people could be confused. She loves that shirt though, so I'll just have to be sure she wears pink pants with it next time.

Well, off to bed now. Both of my angels are sleeping, so I am going to catch up on some sleep too! Love to all, and thanks for continuing to check on little Taylor's progress. We are enjoying the calm that the last few days have brought us. While we know that there are additional tough phases to come, it is good to soak in some of the more pleasant times! Take care, and we'll post more tomorrow.

Love, Kim, Rob, Taylor and Alex

February 25, 2007

As I write this, Taylor and Grandma are putting together a puzzle, and there is lots of laughing going on... Overall, it was a good day- a challenging evening where I felt I was at my wit's end- but then things settled down again, and it was a good day overall.

We started with a visit to the 'little white church' at Bee Ridge Presbyterian. The pastor explained to the congregation during the 8:30 service that Taylor was in town and had asked to come to the 'little white church' (she had requested this during our drive to Sarasota on Friday). Pastor Karl went on to explain that because Taylor could not be around crowds right now due to her Leukemia, he would ask that the congregation forego the standard special prayer request portion of the service that typically happens at the end of each service. This would allow for additional time for Taylor to come in once everyone left. The congregation was more than accommodating, and Pastor Karl and the pianist (Dr. Jonathan) stayed after the morning service to hold a special service for Taylor. When we walked into the little white church, Jonathan began playing 'Jesus Loves Me,' and it just moved me to tears (which I felt bad about because we try so

41

hard to keep from crying in front of Taylor). Taylor looked at me and wiped my face and said 'What is it Mommy?' and I told her 'It's just so beautiful.'

I think what was so beautiful was the overwhelming peace and support I felt being in my home church, holding my daughter and swaying to a beautiful hymn being played for her....and all the time knowing that neither time nor distance has changed the support of the congregation that helped raise me. I hope that everyone at Bee Ridge knows how much today meant to our family. As much as I would have loved to be at the morning service, it's just not possible right now. As soon as Taylor is allowed to attend, we will. During our special service this morning, Pastor Karl also prayed with us and reinforced that God will help support us through this ordeal.

Following church, we headed out to the beach where we had a picnic with Great Grandma, Great Grandpa, Grandma, Grandpa and Alex. We also brought our pails and shovels to play in the sand. Taylor loved the beach, and even ran back and forth in the water. I explained to her that the salt water is so good for any cuts and boo-boos that she has. I think every child that grew up near the ocean / gulf had parents or grandparents that convinced them that the salt water could cure anything. If it could cure cancer, I would have dipped her whole body in today! At a minimum though, I had her wash her hands real good in the gulf...in hopes that it will continue the healing of her fingers (which have been a battle for the past month). She did lots of walking at the beach, including trips down to the water and back to our blanket to get the water for her pails. All of this exercise is so good for her legs, and will hopefully proactively prevent issues with weakening of the muscles.

Well, I know I promised more pictures tonight, but it will most likely be tomorrow. Love to everyone, and I will keep you posted on her progress tomorrow.

Love, Kim, Rob, Taylor and Alex

February 26, 2007

Today was a special day- Grandpa's 60th birthday. Aunt Carol, Uncle Buddy and Kelly came over for dinner, and we celebrated with a spaghetti dinner and cake. We had 'Lightning McQueen' plates, cups, and hats, and Taylor put all of the candles on the cake. Happy Birthday to Grandpa!

It was an okay day overall, although there were quite a few tantrums. There is a balance between attributing tantrums to medicine versus being 3 years old, so it can be tough to discern what the root of the tantrum is at that time. It just so happened that Rob would call in the midst of each of these tantrums, so I'm sure he thinks that today was a total nightmare...it wasn't, just bad timing with calls.

She took her medicine just fine today. It is nice only having the one medicine to take (one time per day too!) She continued to be very active, including wanting to walk down to the pond again to feed the ducks. We are really trying to encourage all of the walking that we can. She would love to go out to the beach again; however, the weather hasn't been cooperating so well- high chances for rain. So, maybe it will hold off long enough tomorrow to get her out there for a little bit.

I have to make tonight's update short as I hear Alex getting fussy, and need to go check on her. Grandpa is uploading the pictures from the past few days, so we will have them to upload shortly. Love to all, and thanks again for all of your guestbook entries. We read them every day....

Love, Kim, Rob, Taylor and Alex

February 27, 2007

Taylor had a great day today....still some tantrums, but overall, we continue to be amazed at how she is doing. She rode her bike for a while again, and she wanted to go back to the beach today. I was more than happy to take her, as we want

43

her to spend as much time outside as possible. She was good about putting sunscreen on her scalp so it didn't get burned and she also found a hat in Grandma's drawer that she likes, so she brought that too.

She played with her buckets and shovels, and played in the water, and she showed me how she was putting water on the boo-boos on her arm so they would get better. I explained to her that if we were to take a boat, we could find Daddy in Panacea. She thought that was pretty neat, although she wants to see it on a map.

She spent some time today looking in the mirror at her 'new buddy' (i.e., the site where her port is). She just spent a lot of time looking at where it was, and pointing to it. I'm sure that she is trying to get used to all of the changes going on.

We are getting ready to go back to Gainesville this Thursday for her clinic visit and lumbar puncture / chemo treatments on Friday. It's becoming pretty routine now- even for Taylor. She has been playing with chemo duck a good bit, and told me last night that she was giving him his 'Decadron' (hope I spelled that right). It made me chuckle that she actually used the proper name of the medicine as opposed to saying 'I'm giving chemo duck his yucky medicine now.' We are realizing that she picks up on the terminology just as we do....

Well, off to bed soon, but I am posting some of her latest pictures tonight. Take care, and we'll keep you posted on the outcomes of her Gainesville visit.

Love, Kim, Rob, Taylor and Alex

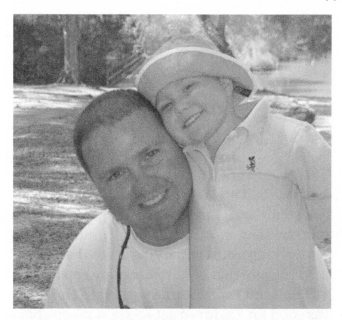

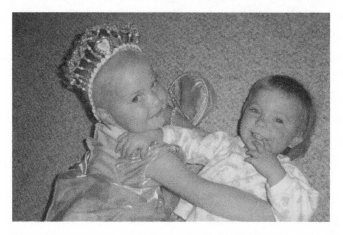

SPRING 2007

Another amazing day...We made another trip to the beach today for a picnic and I can't say enough about how good that walking in the sand must be for her legs! I know that I get tired after walking from the parking lot to the water through the sand, so I'm sure that her little legs are getting good exercise. Miss Ellen and Tanner came with us to the beach today, and it was good for Taylor to get to see someone her age and get to socialize a little bit. Taylor was pretty shy, and still clung pretty tight to Mommy, but I think she liked the idea of having someone at the beach with her that was her age. She also brought Germy to the beach for a visit. She wanted him to see the sand.

She was good about wearing sunscreen on her head again today. Grandpa found some 'spray-on' sunscreen, so we used that and pretended it was hair spray. It seemed to work just fine. I don't know of a great way to help her come to terms with all of the changes going on with her body (i.e., her hair, her up and down weight, etc., the incision line from her port)- but I can tell that she is definitely noticing and focused on them at times. She isn't focused on the changes all of the time, but when she stops to think about it, she'll ask to look in the mirror and just rub her hand over the incision line from her port or just pull more clumps of hair out with her hand...and not know whether it is funny or sad. I think when she is busy riding her bike or marching through the sand, she is too distracted to think about it, so that is probably good. Although, I will add this to the list of questions for the staff at clinic...because she is obviously thinking about these changes sometimes, and I don't want her to feel bad about any of them.

The water weight is continuing to come off. We spend a lot of time running to the potty at the moment, but let me tell you- we've had some of our best conversations there over the past few weeks. It gives you time to talk if nothing else. Her face is less puffy, and she is able to breathe easier lately. It doesn't seem as labored as it was just a week or so ago. She can bend over and pick up things again too, which was very tough for her a little bit ago.

Well, we will be packing in the morning and will get ready to head to Gainesville for our weekly clinic visit and LP / chemo treatment. Assuming all goes well, we will be in Tallahassee again on Friday night. Keeping our fingers crossed that her blood counts continue to come up. I was looking at the report from last week that showed her white blood cell count at 4.5. Normal range starts at 6.0, so hopefully it has continued to climb closer to that...To put it in perspective, she was at 1.3 last month, so she is already making good strides.

Well, love to all, and thanks for checking in on Miss Taylor. She continues to be strong through this, and we are just so proud of her. We'll post some results from clinic as soon as we have them!

March 2, 2007

And we are back from Gainesville! We were there on Thursday and Friday this week. Thursday's clinic visit went well, and she did really well when the nurses accessed her port- no tears! Her ANC (blood count calculation) was 1104 which is in the right range, even though it was lower than last week. I asked the doctor if we should be concerned about that, but she said that it is very normal, as the ANC will be lower as she gets further out from taking the steroids. I really hadn't thought about it that way...because with other illnesses, you would assume that as you get further away from the diagnosis and get further along with medicine that you would get better with each passing day. She is getting better, but the doctor reminded me that the chemotherapy kills the bad cells and the good cells, and that her blood counts will fluctuate along the way. She told me not to be surprised when the ANC goes below 500 again. It will happen, so we have to continue to be careful about exposure to illness. All that said, the doctor was very happy to see how active and happy Taylor was. We explained to her that she had a lot of activity and exercise this week, and that 'Consolidation' feels like night and day compared to 'Induction.' The doctor then reminded me that the steroids will be back at some point, but we don't have to take them right now.

Thursday night was a little tough, as Taylor started crying about pain in her 'buddy' (i.e., her port). We were having dinner, and in mid-sentence, she stopped talking, started crying and said 'It hurts! It hurts!' She couldn't give me specifics except for the fact that it hurt when she pressed on it, but I was worried about it (since this didn't happen last week), so we called the on-call doctor. He explained that it may be pain due to accessing the port, but that they could confirm that during her LP procedure on Friday. When we arrived this morning to the hospital, the pain worsened when they started to give her fluids. During the procedure, they were able to identify that the needle had become dislodged. A separate, but concerning problem was that the port was not allowing the nurses to draw back anything (e.g., blood for blood draws). This led to additional tests today, including a trip to radiology for flow analysis. They injected her with some radioactive dye to watch how it flowed through the port. They quickly identified that there was a blockage at the end of the port due to a film forming over it (her body was doing this naturally- almost if it was fighting an infection). Later this afternoon, they sent us to clinic to have some TPA injected into the port. This is a thinning medicine that helps to get rid of clots. This was effective in helping her port get 'unclogged,' and the nurses were able to draw back from the port. We were happy with the outcome; however, we will still have an additional consult with pediatric surgery next week to see if she needs a new port. The hope is that the TPA is not just a short-term fix, but that will play out by the time we are back in clinic next week. We didn't anticipate it to be a long day, but it was....but that was okay. I'd rather figure out any issues while we are still in Gainesville, as opposed to being 2 hours away.

Taylor has enjoyed being home this evening, and we are hoping to ride our bike some more tomorrow. I hope everyone has a good weekend, and we will keep you updated on how she continues to progress!

Love, Rob, Kim, Taylor and Alex

March 4, 2007

It has been a great weekend overall. Taylor has spent some time riding her bike and playing with friends outside, and then made a trip to the coast today to see 'Daddy's boats' (that is what she calls the boats at Freedom Boat Club). We are very quick to accommodate any outside activity, even if it means driving an hour to be outside (i.e., the trip to see the boats). She has also been doing a ton of puzzles. I really am amazed at how she will spend the time concentrating on her puzzles and figuring them out. I feel like I am learning things about her through this experience...not just that she likes puzzles, but things about her personality too. For example, when we were in 'Induction,' she was having to take several medications twice per day. The nurses had initially told us that they typically gave the steroids last each time because it tasted so bad. We started out this way, but Taylor very quickly pushed to take that medicine first each time. She always just wanted to get the bad stuff out of the way first.

2 weeks ago, I thought I would never make the following statement: I am actually worried that she is not eating enough. We have noticed (especially over the past 2 days) that she has to be reminded (and strongly encouraged) to eat. She did have little bits to eat throughout the day today, but what an interesting contrast to just a week or so ago.

Her daddy reminds me that she is drinking plenty throughout the day and that she is staying hydrated. Additionally, she still appears to have plenty of energy. She is taking a nap during the day- usually for an hour or so, and has resumed sleeping through the night. That was an extremely hard part of the 'Induction' period- minimal sleep for Taylor or Mommy or Daddy. Selfishly, she was a good sleeper at night prior to this diagnosis, and her daddy and I had gotten pretty used to that. Other than eating very little, the only other challenge she seems to be having right now is that her arms are really itchy. There is no rash or visible irritation, but she just scratches a lot. Just another question to ask this week when we are in Gainesville.

Rob and I had the chance to go out to dinner last night while Grandma watched the
girls. I think we both make a conscious effort to try and talk about other topics, but that's not even realistic. The topic of conversation always comes back to Taylor's diagnosis, our hopes and/or fears associated with it, and what the current questions for the doctors will be this week. One conclusion I think we've come to is that there will never be an 'end to the worrying.' We have asked ourselves several times 'When will we be able to stop worrying about the cancer? When will we know that she is okay?' And then we remind ourselves that you always hear parents say that you never stop worrying about your kids- no matter how old they get. I guess this will just put all of the crazy things we'll worry about with her teenage years in perspective as she grows up.

She is sleeping right now, so I should probably get some sleep myself. Thank you so much to everyone who keeps checking in on us. It may be a while yet, but we will get to resume normal visits / socializing at some point I'm sure. The support that everyone has shown means so much, and I just wish we could see everyone right now. Take care, and we'll keep you posted on her progress this week.

March 6, 2007

Today was a good day, with the exception of a couple of breakdowns...but today was also the day where we've attempted to resume our 'old' routine. Up until tonight, Taylor was getting a bath in the morning, but we've resumed bath time at night, playing upstairs, and then reading books to go to bed. Prior to now, and especially during Induction, it seemed as if she was the 'Energizer bunny' (due to steroids, there was little sleep)- so much of the evening was spent downstairs watching movies, playing games...hoping that eventually she would tire out for bedtime. We didn't want her to get too far away from her normal routine, although it has been hard to date. Another change we made today was moving the time she takes her medicine to be 'before dinner.' If she waits until after dinner, we need to wait 2 hours; hence the later bedtimes the past week....so today she took it at 5:00. I am happy to say that it is 8 p.m. and both children are sleeping. It has been too long since we've had that happen!

I am anxious about her trip to Gainesville this week, as we are curious as to what her blood counts will be. Last week, while her ANC was 1104, her hematocrit was 23. If this falls below 20, she will need another transfusion. It will most likely happen sooner or later, but it is just interesting to me how the counts will fluctuate as we continue this experience. She is being a strong little girl this week, and continues to have a lot of energy. She spent a lot of time riding her bike today and playing outside.

We did want to thank Dr. Sue Byrne for fixing Rob's tooth

today! Unfortunately, he broke a tooth the other night, and Sue was able to see him today to get it fixed up...Taylor was very interested as to whether Daddy had to get any 'pokes' to get his tooth fixed today. He told her he did, but that he remembered how brave she was, so he didn't cry. She also wanted to see if he had to take any spicy medicine...

We will keep everyone posted on this week's trip to Gainesville. We are hopeful that the issues with Taylor's port have resolved themselves; however, we do have an appointment scheduled with the pediatric surgeon on Thursday to discuss.

Take care, and thank you again for checking in on little Taylor...

Love, Rob, Kim, Taylor and Alex

March 7, 2007

Another good day in terms of exercise and routine. She spent time today playing at the park with and then time outside playing and running this evening. We did medicine before dinner again tonight, which meant bath time and bedtime went great again tonight. Today was a big day in terms of playing with friends (all of which were free from colds!). Taylor misses school and her friends so much. To the extent that we can (and in short doses), I'm happy that we can play outside with friends. She hasn't seem overly tired from it, and it has been good for her in terms of playing in the fresh air and getting exercise. Her legs are continuing to remain strong, so we are very happy. Abbie, one of her friends, rubbed her head tonight and told her that "she liked her hair now...it's nice and fuzzy." Taylor just smiled.

She does head to clinic in the morning, so we will have a better sense of what her blood counts are. Trending from the past 2 weeks, and the fact that she is further out from the steroids would tell me that her counts will most likely be lower, but we won't make that assumption just yet. Like the doctor said last week- even though her hematocrit was low, she is still exhibiting amazing energy, and seems to be doing great. We do hope that everything with her port is okay. Between the consult with the surgeon tomorrow and the fact that they will try to draw labs via the port tomorrow, I'm sure we will know soon enough!

She will have another lumbar puncture this Friday, and then should be home Friday afternoon (assuming all is well). We will post an update from clinic tomorrow, and thank everyone for their thoughts and prayers.

Love, Kim, Rob, Taylor and Alex

March 8, 2007

Rob and Taylor are in Gainesville tonight, and he said that it was a great day at clinic. The nurses were able to access her port and draw labs from it (so there were no issues with it being 'clogged' this week). That was great news, and eliminated the need (at least for now) to have a follow-up consult with the pediatric surgeon regarding the possibility of a new port. Rob said that Taylor didn't even flinch when Nurse Amy accessed her port. We are so proud of how brave she is...

Her ANC (blood count calculation) was 1120 (up from last week's count of 1104)! In my previous journal entry, I was already assuming that the counts would drop based on trends from the past couple of weeks....but then I remembered that there is not an 'MD' after my name... The doctor did explain to Rob that Taylor's white blood cell counts have dropped from 4.5 to 2.8, but that her neutrophils were up (resulting in the 1120 ANC). The doctor also went on to explain that they need Taylor's ANC to stay between 500 and 1500 right now, and that if it goes outside of that range that they will adjust her medication dosages to bring it back into that range. I don't quite understand why that is, so we do want to follow up with them to better understand it. At the end of the day, they are the experts in this area, so there must be a good reason that the range is in place!

All of the Gator fans out there will appreciate this next part: Taylor had a big field trip with her Daddy today to 'The Swamp.' You know her Daddy must love her to take her on a special field trip there...but she requested it this past week. We were driving by the stadium last week during our trip to clinic, and she asked me if we could go see the 'Gator Place' (i.e., the football field). She explained to me that it is 'an outside place, and I won't have to wear my mask.' I would have loved to take her last week, but because it was starting to get dark outside at that point, I explained that we would need to wait until our next visit to Gainesville. She has been anticipating her visit to The Swamp all week. Rob said she ran all over the stadium and had a great time. Upon their return to Tallahassee, I'm sure a trip to Doak Campbell will be quick to follow.

She will have her LP procedure in the morning, and assuming everything is okay, she will be on the road back to Tallahassee tomorrow. Alex and I had a good day in Tallahassee playing, running errands and getting things done around the house. It was good to have some Alex and Mommy time, and I'm sure Rob was happy to be with Taylor today.

The LP tomorrow is the last one we'll have for a bit. Next week, she will just have clinic visit, and then the doctors will be focused on assessing whether she is ready for the next phase called 'Standard Interim Maintenance.' That phase will reintroduce steroids for 5 days at a time, along with other new medications. Following the Standard Interim Maintenance phase, she will move into 'Delayed Intensification' which we understand will be very similar to the 'Induction' period. It is good for us to look ahead and try to be prepared, but for now- we will focus on finishing out 'Consolidation,' and enjoying the fact that it seems to be a little easier on Taylor's little body and spirit.

Love to all, and we will keep you posted on her LP tomorrow.

Love, Rob, Kim, Taylor and Alex

March 9, 2007

The LP today went fine. She was in and out of the procedure and back in Tallahassee by mid-day. Her port worked just fine this week which was a blessing. She spent time playing outside when she got home, and even rode along with me to the hairdresser. Her school is right next door to the strip mall where the salon is, and the 'big kid' playground backs up to the strip mall. When we got out of the car, she noticed that her class was outside playing, so she ran up to the fence and started shouting to her friends and teachers. They all ran over to see her. At first she was excited, and then she got a little overwhelmed and ran to Grandma....and then Grandma reminded her that her friends missed her a lot too, and that is why they were all wanting to talk to her at the same time...so she ran back to see them. Overall, it has been amazing to me how kids react with questions. They ask a question such as 'Why does Taylor have short hair now?' You give them an answer, and then they move on. They don't dwell.

Her friends saw the mask we were holding, and wanted to know what it was. Taylor showed her friends how she puts the mask on and can make 'fishy lip' faces underneath it and no one can tell. She blew kisses to everyone when we left, and told us in the car how much she misses everyone. I told her that she'll see them again real soon.

She was pretty tired tonight after dinner, and fell asleep right after she ate. Bath time will have to wait until morning time, but that is okay...she needs her sleep. She has been such a trooper, and we are very proud of her. She made us laugh tonight when she said she didn't need applesauce or the pill crusher for her evening medicine- she just took the pill, chewed it up and swallowed it. She ended up taking a couple of bites of applesauce after she chewed it up, but only because I encouraged her too. I figured the medicine had to leave a bad taste in her mouth, and that the applesauce would at least make that go away. She just continues to amaze us.

Well, we hope everyone has a great weekend. We will keep you posted on her progress this week and her clinic visit as well. Thank you again for your notes of encouragement. We really appreciate them, and look forward to reading them every day.

March 10, 2007

Another day of lots of outside play. We spent a good bit of time at the park this afternoon, and only left because it started to get too crowded. Taylor's friend Jenna came over to play this afternoon too. Taylor was so excited to have her come and play. When she saw all of her friends at school yesterday, she wanted to have everyone over to play. I told her we'll have to do that slowly...All of the outside play must have made her pretty tired though. I finally convinced her it was time to head inside for dinner when I realized it was almost 7:00. While I was making her dinner, she fell asleep on the couch. At first, I tried waking her up for dinner and bath, but she was out. So, instead I just carried her up to bed and told myself that she is just getting on the right clock for Daylight Savings Time.

For those of you who have children or loved ones battling Leukemia and have forwarded us links to your websites, Rob and I have appreciated your supportive words. To a certain extent, I think I try to focus on nothing but a full recovery, and I think reading through everyone's websites forces Rob and I to keep a more realistic perspective. Part of me would like to block out anything that even slightly indicates that there will be anything unexpected (i.e., more hospital admissions, infections, side effects to chemo, relapses), but I guess deep down I know that I should be more realistic. Having said all of that, if I consider everything that can happen, there would be no way to stay positive.

Rob in particular has been good about researching and reading through other websites of families that have children diagnosed with ALL, and he reminds me that there is a long road ahead. One website in particular struck me hard today- Mackenzie Johnson's: (http://www.caringbridge.org/il/mackenzie/index.htm). Mackenzie's Leukemia has relapsed twice over the course of her treatment, even though she showed remission early on. She is now looking for a bone marrow donor. Her family is asking folks to write the Oprah Winfrey show as Oprah is granting 1 wish to someone in the Chicago area. Mackenzie's wish is to find a bone marrow donor, and her family is asking Oprah to get the word out and raise awareness with hopes of finding a potential donor. I wrote my letter to Oprah today. It took maybe 5 minutes to complete. If you have some time today, just click on the following link and ask Oprah to consider Mackenzie's wish as the one to be chosen.(https://www.oprah.com/plugger/templates/BeOnTheShow.jhtml?action=respond&plugId =256400006)

Reading her site also made me realize that I haven't even taken the step yet to get tested to be a potential bone marrow donor. Hopefully, this is not a procedure that

Taylor will need; but there may be someone, someday who could use my marrow, so why not just go ahead and get registered? That is something to put on my to-do list and get done.

Well, we thank you again for your caring words and prayers. We'll post more tomorrow....

Love, Kim, Rob, Taylor and Alex

March 12, 2007

As Rob and I have said in previous updates, we thank everyone for the outpouring of support. Friends, family, and the community have just been amazing in reaching out to us to see what would be helpful as Taylor progresses through her treatment. I also wanted to send thank yous out tonight to fire departments across the state, including Jefferson County. Mr. Dexter stopped by to see Taylor the other day and brought her a special gift from the fire department out there...Your generosity is so appreciated.

We spent lots of outside time today, including a picnic on the pontoon boat. Rob had a meeting down at the coast today, so the girls and I tagged along to find 'more outside things' to do! Taylor and Alex had a great time looking for turtles, fishies, and birds on our trip. They each took turns trying to drive the boat with Daddy too. Rob brought a fishing pole with him so that he and Taylor could try to catch some fish- not much luck today, but we'll head out again to try at some point. When we got back to town, we headed to the park for a little bit to get some time on the playground. Once it got crowded though, it was time to head home. She is keeping her energy up, and playing hard throughout the day. While I'm not sure if there is any 'medical' justification for it, I've got to believe that it is some of the best medicine for her.

With the exception of some frustrating tantrums, things are going really well right now. She is taking her medicine without any issue, and is getting good sleep at night. I know that in subsequent weeks (as soon as next week) that the steroids will be back and that some of these things will change, but we'll deal with that when it happens.

Per my posting the other night, I will check with the doctors this week to understand the general process for being tested to be a bone marrow donor. When I find out, I will post it in the journal update...Thanks to everyone for your postings. We'll keep you posted on her progress this week and her upcoming clinic visit...

March 13, 2007

Today was a good day overall, including a picnic and playtime at the park. We are still having some frustrating tantrums; however, I am sure that part of it is being 3, and part of it is that she is just continuing to test her limits. Her daddy and I are doing our best to reinforce routine and structure, and will just need to keep doing so. On the flip side, there are so many good times during the day, and in spite of everything going on- it is great to see Taylor and Alex have so much time together during the day. Taylor is very excited about teaching her little sister lots of things. Today, she helped her perfect 'brushing her teeth.' This afternoon, she was intent on teaching Alex how to drive the 'Barbie Jeep.' I tried explaining that Alex's feet can't reach the pedals yet, so Taylor just sat in the passenger seat and handled the steering wheel and the gas pedal while Alex sat in the driver's seat and just laughed.

Granny (the wonderful lady who watched Taylor until she was 2....and up until recently, Alex too!) baked some yummy cookies for Taylor today, and we went by this evening to visit. Taylor and Alex were excited to see Granny, and Taylor was very happy that Granny promised to make her more cookies! The change of scenery was good for the girls, and I explained to Granny that I'm pretty sure that Taylor is bored with just having Rob and I as playmates by now....Each day Taylor asks me if it is a 'school day' and whether any of her friends are free to play. She is pretty bummed when I tell her it is a 'school day,' but that she is not able to go just yet. As much as she loves to go to the park, she misses her friends at school a lot!

All in all, we continue to take each day as it comes, and we are very happy about how she is progressing through the treatment. We pray that she will continue to respond to the treatment and that the cancer cells stay away...Her clinic visit is coming up on this Thursday, so hopefully we will have some additional insight into the next phase of treatment that will be coming up in the next week or so.

Love to everyone, and thank you so much to Dawn and everyone who dug deeper into the bone marrow donor info. I will also talk to Taylor's doctors about it this week.

Love, Rob, Kim, Taylor and Alex

March 14, 2007

Today was kind of a tough day, for no other reason than Taylor threw a lot of fits today. By this evening, she was in a much better mood, and was happy to see her daddy when he got home from the fire station. She knows she is headed to clinic tomorrow, and I do think she starts to get a little anxious about it (and is also another reason that probably factors into her acting out-but that may also be an excuse I try to tell myself too!). We try not to focus too much on clinic ahead of time, but she is aware that it is coming up at some point. Having said all of that, she was doing a lot of 'role playing' with her dolls today. She told me that her baby doll was having a 'procedure' done today, and that she needed to go outside and play in the waiting room while the doctors did the procedure. She set her baby doll up in the family room with all sorts of 'doctor tools' around her (which happened to include an FM modulator that she pulled off of the shelf...but she said it was the tube for the baby's medicine). She told me that her baby didn't have a port, so she would need to get a 'poke.' She told the baby that it would be okay, and that she would be outside in the waiting room.

While she doesn't do a 'procedure' every day on one of her dolls, it is pretty standard for her to do some sort of role playing at least once each day. That is why her chemo duck comes in so handy. It was such a great idea for the child life specialist to give her that duck. She has even tried showing Alex how to attach the syringe to chemo duck's port. At a minimum, I guess she is using the role playing to try to process everything that is happening to her. It is a balance because sometimes it is mildly comical while at the same time heartbreaking. Alex sneezed yesterday, and Taylor got really concerned. She asked me if Alex had 'cancer germs,' and I told her that I thought she was okay. She told me that we could take her to the doctors if we needed to.

Well, we are off to Gainesville in the morning. It is supposed to be a day trip, so the goal is to come home without having to unpack our suitcase! Tomorrow may be a little bit of a tough visit for her, as she will have to get 'a poke' (i.e., a needle stick to get her labs drawn). She has gotten used to having the blood drawn from her buddy, which doesn't cause her any pain. She gets pretty nervous about 'pokes,' but this will be one of many to come I'm sure...I know she will be fine, and will do the best that I can to keep her distracted / thinking happy thoughts, etc. while they do the needle stick.

We'll post an update tomorrow night on the results from clinic, and thank you again for your support and prayers.

Love, Rob, Kim, Taylor and Alex

March 16, 2007

Taylor's clinic visit went great yesterday. Her counts were over 1500, and it was amazing to look at her lab sheet and see that her platelet count, her hemoglobin, and her hematocrit were all within the normal levels. Her white blood cell count was 3.2, which continues to be lower than the normal range (which starts at 6.0), but the doctors are comfortable with her overall ANC of 1500. Her energy has been great, and the doctors are happy with her progress. Dr. Hunger explained that she will begin Standard Interim Maintenance next Thursday. This will mean resuming steroids, but only for 5-day increments. She will also be on some additional medicines, including new oral and IV chemotherapy medicines, but I am happy to think that she is well enough to progress to the next phase. Dr. Hunger did shed some light on her current medication (the 6-MP). He asked that Taylor not chew it, but instead try to swallow it in pieces...or the whole thing. So, we will be back to cutting it in pieces to put in the applesauce. He also explained that research has shown that children who take the medicine at night (versus in the morning) are less likely to relapse. Having said that, Rob and I are also pushing her medicine back from taking it in early evening to right before bedtime. About a week or so ago, we had started giving it before dinner- now, she will get it closer to 8 p.m. I beat myself up for a while last night about whether or not we've hurt her progress by having her taking it earlier the past week or so...but then figured we can't change that now, so we'll move forward with right before bedtime.

Dr. Hunger said there will be some tough times with the delayed intensification phase (which will follow Standard Interim Maintenance), but that we will have 2 months until that comes. I think the 'tough times' he is referring to is the 21-day stint of steroids. I also asked him about her appetite, as she is never hungry now! While she is eating a decent amount during the day, it is only because we are harping on it all day long. Having the steroids back next week may be helpful in that area, so I will try to see the silver lining in that.

During our visit yesterday, Nurse Amy was able to draw the blood by accessing Taylor's port, so there was no need for a lab draw (i.e., the needle poke that she was so dreading). She didn't flinch during the access (god bless the numbing cream that we have the prescription for!), and even helped flush the line with Saline and Heparin when Nurse Amy was done. The nurses are amazing about how they let the kids help. Taylor was able to help her get the blood in the tubes to go the lab...which made her feel like such a big helper. She laughed and played with the nurses, and told me she'd just like to stay there for a while. It is great to see her anxiety about clinic getting better and better. We'll head back to clinic next week, but it appears that we will only have to have 1 LP over the next 8 weeks.

As I write this, we are watching the Wiggles. I can officially say that I have learned all of the words to 'Big Red Car' and 'Fruit Salad.' The ability to be home with both Taylor and Alex has been great, and Rob and I will continue to balance that and work as she continues treatment. I know that she will be excited to get back to school and her friends, but she will most likely be home full time until the Fall.

Well, we hope everyone has a great weekend. We'll keep you posted, and are hopeful for another good week. Love, Rob, Kim, Taylor and Alex

March 18, 2007

Another good weekend overall...the girls wore their green on St. Patrick's Day, and went to visit Daddy at the fire station (and brought cookies). Today we were all able to spend time together playing. We have adjusted Taylor's medicine schedule, so it does mean for a later bedtime, but whatever it takes is okay with us! She doesn't mind getting to come downstairs after bath time to watch a movie before medicine and bedtime, so that works out okay...

Our big event this weekend was eating out at a restaurant for the first time in 2 months. There is a little pizzeria near us with an outside deck. It wasn't crowded on Friday night, so we took the opportunity to eat there. Taylor was so excited. She didn't want to leave! Since then, she is naming every-place she can that has an 'outside place' to eat. When we were driving around town today, she was on the look-out for more places to eat outside.

Things are going well, but I will admit that sometimes it gets so draining. Rob and I were talking over dinner tonight, and can't believe that we are only 2 months into this. 2 1/2 years seems very far off...and to know that her little body will have to continue with such intense treatment just breaks your heart at times. Having said that- how blessed are we that we are only 2 months into this and that she is already in remission? What an amazing thing.

We will keep you posted on her week. She has requested to go back to 'The Swamp' again this week during her trip to Gainesville...so I'll have to break that to her Daddy. We will resume steroids later this week, so I am praying for the strength and patience that we will need.

Love to all....and thank you for everything.

March 20th- so we are officially 2 months into her treatment. I read somewhere that you will never forget your child's date of diagnosis. I can understand that.

Yesterday was a good day overall. We ate at another outside place, although you find yourself constantly wiping / disinfecting everything in sight. It is still worth it though because she had a great time, and she ate relatively well considering her lower appetite recently. Rob reminds me that she will resume her steroids on Thursday, so I'm sure her appetite will spike back up again. The highlight of yesterday was watching 'Dancing with the Stars' with Taylor. She dressed up in her sunglasses, a hooded towel over her pajamas, and a necklace and danced each time one of the couples was dancing. It was adorable. (and it kept her up late enough to take her 6-MP 2 hours after she finished eating, and then straight to bed!)

Alex woke up this morning, and I thought I heard some sniffles, so I will need to keep an eye on her. Hopefully, it was just from waking up this morning and will go away. Maybe it's her teeth or maybe it's nothing, but I can't even explain how scary the thought of one of us being sick is. A common cold could put Taylor back in the hospital, so it is so important for the four of us to stay healthy right now.

I wanted to thank the Gendusas for the yummy meals they put together for us. It is so appreciated, and takes one more task out of the mix for the day! Thank you so much!

I did take pictures of her princess room and will get those uploaded tonight...Love to all, and we'll write more later.

Love, Rob, Kim, Taylor and Alex

We are getting ready to head back to Gainesville in the morning. Aunt Debbie is coming to clinic with us tomorrow, so Taylor is excited. Tomorrow she will have her blood counts done as well as begin the next phase of treatment (standard interim maintenance). She will receive additional chemotherapy treatments via her 'buddy' tomorrow while we are at clinic, but overall, it is anticipated to be a day trip. We will pack our bag, but plan not to unpack while we are there!

We had a wonderful day today. Taylor's friend, Haley, invited her down to St. Teresa to go to the beach. We had a really nice time playing on the beach, looking for shells, and splashing in the water. Thank you so much to the Knox family for having us down to visit today. When we started treatment, one of the counselors told me to work with Taylor to find a 'happy place' she could think of to calm her down if she got scared. Taylor has told us that Haley's beach house is her 'happy place' that she thinks of...It is really sweet to think that she has such good memories of a place she has visited before!

Well, off to bed to get some rest, and promises to update more when we get back from clinic. I pray that the steroids are easier on her little body this time around, but know that she is a strong little girl. Love to all, and we'll post more shortly...

Love, Rob, Kim, Taylor and Alex

March 23, 2007

Well we knew she was brave- but who knew she was brave enough to waltz into the Swamp wearing her FSU cheerleader outfit! She asked to wear her cheerleader outfit yesterday down to clinic, and her treat for being so good at clinic was to visit the Swamp again...She took Aunt Debbie, Mommy, and Alex to visit it this time. Daddy was at the fire station, but she said she will bring him again next time.

Her clinic visit went great yesterday (once we got there that is). Getting in the car in Tallahassee is a nightmare. She will be okay, and then she starts yelling, screaming, kicking, and scratching (as the onlookers at the Shell Gas Station witnessed yesterday), and says that she is not going on the interstate. It is frustrating, because you have no choice but to be strong and force her into the car, but it breaks your heart to have to do it. Once she gets to clinic though, she runs in and can't wait to see all of the nurses. Taylor was very excited to show Aunt Debbie all about clinic and what she does there. She did great through her weigh-in / height / temperature and blood pressure, and she didn't even want me to sit near her- she wanted to do it all by herself. There are always plenty of hugs for Miss Donna, Miss Amy, and Miss Jenna...Mr. Dax wasn't there yesterday, but Taylor told me she'll get to see him next time. Taylor did great when they accessed her port to draw blood, and her port didn't give the nurses any issues (in terms of being 'clogged up' or anything). She received additional chemo through her buddy yesterday, and we began her new phase called 'Standard Interim Maintenance.' This meant resuming the steroids this morning, and adding a new weekly chemo set of pills to her regimen (Methotrexate). She will continue to take the 6-MP daily and the steroids daily, and the new chemo pill is only taken once per week. She will also continue her Septra (a strong antibiotic) 3 days per week. All of that said, her medicines are becoming pretty routine for us, and Dr. Hunger explained that this is the same set of medicine she will be on during her 'Maintenance' period. He explained that the next 8 weeks should give us a preview of what the long term 'Maintenance' phase will be like.

He also explained that for now she has additional restrictions lifted regarding activities. With good judgement by Mom and Dad, we can go eat inside at a restaurant, and go to movie theaters, etc. He explained that from mid-May to mid-July will be her highest risk period for infection (due to the chemo treatment being stronger during 'delayed intensification'), so he said to try to enjoy as much as we can with normal activities during this phase. Her ANC was 1650 yesterday, so that was also reassuring. We are very happy that she is continuing to progress, and Dr. Hunger explained that her end of treatment will be 2 years from the start of 'Standard Interim Maintenance' (i.e., 2 years from yesterday). That is still a long way off, and a lot of medicine on her little body, but I know that we can get through this together. In a few years, we hope to look back on it all as a memory. I won't say a bad memory, because I truly believe there are some good life lessons we are learning / experiencing as a result of it, but a memory just the same. Love to all, and we'll keep you posted on her progress this week!

Love, Rob, Kim, Taylor and Alex

March 25, 2007

It has been a good weekend so far. Today is Day 3 of steroids for this month, and it is going better than we thought it would. One trick that has helped was putting her Decadron (the steroids) in juice. I happened to read that the medicine could be put in juice to mask the taste, but I called Taylor's doctors to make sure they were okay with it. They said it would be fine to do that, so now that is how we will be giving the 'spicy, yucky' medicine (as Taylor would call it). While I wish we would have known that during the Induction period, I also wouldn't appreciate the benefit of it now I guess...

That isn't to say that there haven't still been challenges with taking her medicine the past few days, but it has been a much better experience overall. We've had later nights the past few nights, as the steroids don't allow her to go to sleep as easily; however, we were pleasantly surprised that she has slept through the night! I know we still have a few days to go on them, but a 5-day stint is definitely different than the 29-day stint we went through in Induction.

As I write this, I am outside with the girls while they are playing. Taylor is driving around in her jeep with her baby dolls, and Alex is playing by the swing. It is so nice to be able to take advantage of the beautiful weather. We're also going to be taking the girls to the FSU / Boston College baseball game this afternoon- another great outside activity!

Grandma is moving up today to help out, and we are so happy. The next 8 weeks should be an easier time on Taylor, but there is still a long way to go, so the help is definitely appreciated. I continue to pray for patience and strength to effectively deal with any situations that arise, and I'll thank all of you every day for the support that you provide us.

Love to all, and we'll keep you posted on her progress this week....

Love, Rob, Kim, Taylor and Alex

March 26, 2007

I am a grown woman, so I should know better than to jinx something by saying in my previous journal entry that 'Taylor was sleeping through the night.' :)

Last night was a little tougher- up a couple times, and trouble sleeping overall. She wouldn't fall asleep until after 11:00, and I was having trouble staying awake with her until she did...which made her even more frustrated. She has been crying since she woke up this morning, and doesn't want anyone around her...Only 2 more days of the steroids this month, so I know that this will soon pass.

All of that aside, yesterday was a great day out at the baseball game. She had a wonderful time, and cheered as loud as she could for the Seminoles. Her daddy had her bring her little broom to the game, and I tried to explain to her that it was because the Seminoles were 'sweeping' Boston College. I think by the end of the game she kinda understood that....but she just thought it was fun to play with. Grandma also arrived to town safely, so we are happy that she is here.

Well, I know things will get better, but today feels like a tough day. I'm sure that will make the week to come feel a little better. Love to all, and we'll write more later.

Love, Rob, Kim, Taylor, and Alex

March 27, 2007

What started out as a tough day yesterday turned into a great day. She felt good enough to play at the park in the afternoon where we played with Madison, Lexi and Miss Lori. Evening time went well as she was excited about 'Dancing With the Stars' coming on (which is no problem to stay up for when she is on these steroids!) As it got later though, you could tell that she was tired, but couldn't rest. It is so frustrating to her, and frustrating for us to watch her feel so tired, but not be able to sleep. Rob was finally able to get her to sleep around 11:00, and we were quick to follow. And Aunt Kim's update was right- I am pitiful when it comes to staying up late! Thankfully, Taylor rested well, and didn't wake up until around 6:00 this morning. Today is the last day of steroids for the next few weeks, but you can see the effects starting to take toll. Her belly is giving her some trouble this morning. We are going to call the doctors about the possibility of her taking some Pepcid (which was prescribed last time, but not this time due to the shorter duration of the steroids). With today being the last day, we may still see some side effects for the next couple of days, but are hoping they will subside by the weekend. Overall, she is doing well though, and we will just take it day by day.

We wanted to thank the Cooksey family for ordering custom bracelets for Taylor. They are purple and say 'Princess Taylor Ann Koegel' on them. Several of the firefighters are wearing them in support of Taylor, and Sarah had a box ready for us to pick up yesterday. Several friends and family members have let us know they are interested in ordering some, so I promise we will have that figured out later today...and will post it to the website. I can't say it enough times- how blessed we are to have support from so many areas and in so many ways. With all that is going on, I would have never found the time to research websites for custom bracelets, but Sarah gets it done! Thanks so much!

Also- a big thank you to the teams that are getting ready for the American Cancer Society's 'Relay for Life' on April 13th. I know that all of you have been focused on encouraging fundraising for cancer research which will not only benefit little Taylor, but so many people. Taylor is very excited about getting to walk around the track as part of the first lap. She is debating whether she would like to walk, ride her scooter, ride her bike, or go in the wagon. My guess is that we will be probably be toting all of these modes of transportation in the minivan that day...

Well, I will sign off for now. It's tough to type with the kids trying to get to the computer :)

Love, Rob, Kim, Taylor and Alex

March 27, 2007

Tonight was her last dose of steroids for the month...so I guess there is approximately a 3 week break before she needs to take them again. She did really well taking her medicine tonight, and she is very excited that she only has to take 1 medicine tomorrow (her 6-MP). I think I've posted this before, but there are mixed emotions of being proud and extremely sad when your 3-year-old can use a pill crusher and mix her own medicine with applesauce (supervised of course, but she is definitely little Miss Independent). She has also wanted to learn how to draw up her various medicines in the syringes too. She is actually much more favorable to taking her medicine when she assists with getting it prepared. I guess that makes sense, so we will do what works.

We had a beautiful moment in the car today when we were driving home from dinner. She said 'Mommy and Grandma- listen to me: Dear God, Thank you for my Mommy, my Daddy, my baby sister Alex, etc......Amen.' (She went through a whole list, I promise she didn't say etc.) I told her that it was a beautiful prayer, and that I thank God for her every day. Then she told me that she is going to be an 'angel up there with the thunder.' My eyes just filled up with tears because it was so innocent and almost frightening to me- like she knew something that we didn't- like she was planning to go to heaven sometime soon. I know I shouldn't think like that, and I know I have no reason to think that everything isn't going to work out just fine- but there are moments of doubt- not in God and his plan for her, but in what we are able to do to keep her here as long as I want her here. I am happy that she wants to hear and learn about God, and I read her bible stories as she is interested to hear. Selfishly though, I hope that God's plan is to keep her here very healthy and for a very long time.

Enough sad thoughts though- she is sleeping peacefully now, and had a great day overall. I am getting ready to go back to work shortly (on a part-time basis), so I will miss being with Taylor and Alex every day, but there will still be a lot of valuable time together- at least 2 days during the week and both weekend days, so there will be a good balance.

Thank you to everyone for checking in on her progress, and thanks so much for your postings in the guestbook. I know that it must be hard sometimes to figure out what to say / post- if anything. Don't worry about what to say- just say anything- even Hi....we love to know you are out there.

Love, Rob, Kim, Taylor and Alex

March 28, 2007

Miss Taylor is sleeping peacefully again...no nap today, but we are pretty sure that is because the steroids are still in her system (but wearing off!) There were some outbursts today. It is so hard to explain how you walk on eggshells, but you just don't know what will start an outburst! It could be that Mommy finished brushing her teeth before Taylor did or that Alex made it down the stairs first, or my favorite: "My food is touching! Throw it all away and make me new food Mommy!!!." I guess some of it can seem comical after the fact...but during an outburst...not so funny...

We spent some time at the park again today, and had a picnic with Grandma for lunch. It is nice to have Mom's help, especially in the evenings when dinner, bath time, bedtime, and medicine time seem to come all at once! The girls are happy she is here, and aren't quite understanding that she is not leaving. Each time she gets in the car, Taylor thinks she is headed to Sarasota, but I've explained that 'she might just be running to the store.' I'm sure that as they see her every day, they will start to understand that she lives here now.

We are hopeful that the steroid effects continue to subside. She is supposed to play at the park tomorrow with one of her friends from school, and she is so excited! Playdates like this keep her motivated about each day's activities, and we also started a 'sticker chart' tonight to help reinforce good behavior. We had read about sticker charts before being helpful (even during steroid treatment), as the stickers are very motivating for most children her age. She even helped me come up with a list of things she should be responsible for on her list...brushing her teeth twice daily, taking her bath, being nice to Alex, no hitting, and helping set the table.

Well, time to sign off for tonight. Time to carry Miss Taylor up to bed, and to take care of some things before going to bed myself. Love to all, and we'll write more tomorrow.

Love, Rob, Kim, Taylor and Alex

March 30, 2007

We've had a great couple of days...time at the park with friends, and a special visit from Miss Garrett from school today. Taylor played with Dawson yesterday at the park, and couldn't stop talking about it last night. Today she met up with Camryn, Carson, and Abbie at the park too. When she got back from the park, Miss Garrett had stopped by to visit. Taylor loves it when Miss Garrett comes to play. I still remember being in the hospital on Day 4 of treatment, and Taylor's eyes just lighting up when Garrett walked in to see her. She talked more that day than any other day that we were at the hospital. Miss Garrett's visit today has been great. She even stayed through Taylor's bath time, and played puzzles afterward...

I am back to work on Monday, and Rob and I will balance time with the kids over the week. Taylor understands that I am going back to work, and that I have lots of 'meetings' to go to. She told me that when I am in meetings, Daddy will stay with her and Alex...and that when I'm not in meetings, Daddy will be at his work at the 'boat station.' (That is what she calls Rob's fire station because they have a boat there). There will never be the perfect time to go back to work, but we are in a period right now where her energy and health seem to be doing well, and are projected to continue to do well over the next 7 weeks. Mid-May to Mid-July may be a different story, so I want to make sure to save time for when I need it the most.

Her energy level continues to be amazing. We've had a couple of issues over the past day in terms of diarrhea and some skin breakdown on her bottom, so we are trying to address the skin breakdown with zinc ointment. This is one of the side effects of her chemo medicine, so we have to watch that very closely. She was very good about putting on the ointment tonight, and we are just passing time this evening until it's time for her nighttime meds...

Love to all, and we will write more tomorrow. Aunt Kathy is driving up to visit this weekend, so Taylor is looking forward to that. We'll write more tomorrow!

Love, Rob, Kim, Taylor and Alex

April 1, 2007

We have had a full weekend! Yesterday, Taylor went to her friend Cade's birthday party. It was the first party she had been able to attend in a while, so she was very excited! It was a superhero party, so she flew around with her cape and pretended to fly....she had an amazing time. It was nice for her to catch up with her friends, and it was great for me to meet some friends that have been praying for us over the past few months. While I had not previously met some of the moms in attendance before, they have gotten to know us through the website...it was so nice to meet everyone in person! Aunt Kathy was in town this weekend, and was so helpful at the party. It took 2 of us to keep up with Taylor and Alex! The girls were happy to spend time with Aunt Kathy this weekend, and are excited that she will be back soon for the Firefighter's Benefit on April 21st. Several of you have asked me for more information about tickets. I promise to check in about that and post more on the website. For now, a link for initial information can be found via http://www.iafflocal2339.org/. Hope to see you there!

Taylor attended church this morning for Palm Sunday, and had a great time singing. The kids got a little antsy near the end of church, so we headed outside to wait for Aunt Kathy. It was perfect timing though because we ran into Father O'Sullivan on our way outside. He and I had a chance to chat about a parish member whose daughter had Leukemia when she was young, and is now 30 years old with children of her own! It helps Rob and I to hear these success stories, and reinforces our hopes for Taylor's progress. I was happy we ran into him this morning!

This weekend was not without several outbursts- some that are so frustrating...so I continue to pray for more patience. I realize I become pretty snappy to those around me when these happen as well (Rob takes the brunt of this unfortunately), so it is a personal goal of mine to get better about that! Going back to work this week will probably give me more patience at night to deal with outbursts (as I will be missing the girls during the day), but I'm sure it is an ongoing process.

We had a surprise visit from a neighbor last night who

brought by some ointment that she said should help with Taylor's skin breakdown...and some Aveeno bath soap that may help as well. I can't tell you how I continue to be touched by the generosity of friends, family, and people we have never met up until now. Thank you, thank you, thank you so much!!!

This week we will head to 'Kids Corner' at our local hospital for Taylor to get some of her bloodwork done. I am interested to know if they will be accessing her port or doing the blood draw via a needle stick, so I want to call tomorrow. This will help give us time to prepare Taylor if necessary (or to understand if we can use some of the special numbing cream on her arm instead!) While I am happy that we can stay in town this week for her bloodwork, it is still a delicate situation when trying to help her get over the possibility of a 'poke.'

Well, I hear Alex waking up from her afternoon nap...so I need to run. Love to all, and we'll update more tomorrow!

Love, Rob, Kim, Taylor, and Alex

April 2, 2007

If I haven't mentioned it before, I have the most amazing husband. I try to remember to tell him that on a regular basis, but I'm sure I don't tell him enough. He gave me such a comfort level about going back to work today. Rob called it the first day of 'Daddy Daycare...' The kids had a blast today with Daddy, and we all had a nice dinner (prepared by Daddy) when I got home from work tonight. Aunt Debbie and Grandma were there for dinner too, so it was extra nice! Rob amazes me with everything he is able to get done during the day. Somehow he was able to get the oil changed in the car, continue with the chores at the house, get Easter Bunny pictures and have plenty of time to play outside today with the kids. I can't imagine being strong through all of this without him. He did mention that he fit in a nap too-I need to watch and learn!

Taylor received a package from Clemson this weekend at Grandma's house. Grandma brought it back with her on her trip back to Tallahassee so Taylor could open it. It is a signed picture from the Clemson Tiger, and he sent along an orange baseball t-shirt for her too. The Tiger picture now has a place of honor on her bedroom dresser.

Taylor had a little bit of an upset tummy today- which resulted in Daddy cleaning the floors as well. It seemed to be an isolated episode though, and she felt better soon after....we don't think it was related to any of her medications because there haven't been any new medications in over a week...so hopefully it was just something she ate that didn't agree with her tummy.

Taylor watched a little bit of 'Dancing with the Stars' before falling asleep tonight. We recorded it so she can watch it later though. We talked to her about her upcoming appointment at Kid's Corner on Thursday. I explained that I talked to the nurse today and that she told me that they could access her buddy for the blood draw if that is what she prefers....There was also the option of a finger stick. We told her that we'll continue to chat about it and that it is her choice. Right now she says she would like them to access her buddy.

Well, love to all, and we'll keep you posted on her progress this week.

April 3, 2007

Another great day with Daddy. Rob and the girls met me for lunch today, so that was a nice treat. After a good day with the girls, it was time for Rob to go on shift, so I just needed to make sure to leave work in time for him to get to the fire station on time. We're working out the kinks to make sure everyone gets where they need to be on time...but I think we're doing okay for Day 2 of being back to work.

Taylor felt really good today- no upset tummy, and in a great mood overall. She ate really well tonight too. As far as her medicine goes, she has learned to take her daily medicine in one big gulp, which impresses me (because her 6-MP is not a tiny pill!)

Rob was noticing that she is a little shaky at times before meal time, so he was a bit concerned about her blood sugar, and wanted to see if the doctors think we should look at that as part of her labs this week. If so, that is something that can be done here in Tallahassee as well, and the results will just be sent to her doctors in Gainesville.

Well, I have some work to get done before heading to bed, so love to all...and we will post more tomorrow!

April 6, 2007

Taylor had a great visit to KidsCorner yesterday here in Tallahassee. She made the choice to have her port accessed instead of getting a finger stick. While the finger stick would have been quicker for her, giving her choices is important too. There are so many times that she does not have choices about what she can and cannot do, so when she can have one-that's great.

Ironically, the nurse that accessed her port yesterday was named 'Nurse Donna' (same as one of Taylor's nurses at clinic), so I think that helped Taylor feel that much more comfortable! She told Nurse Donna that the other Nurse Donna and Nurse Amy let her help when she is at clinic. So, Taylor continued to help with flushing her port, and getting the blood in the vacutainers. Nurse Donna (here in Tallahassee) said that Taylor was a very good helper.

We received some preliminary blood count info from Tallahassee Memorial, but I am still waiting to hear back from Shands to make sure the counts are right. If we calculated it right, Taylor's ANC is 750. While this is down from 2 weeks ago, her hematocrit and hemoglobin were 11 and 34 which is good. Her platelets were over 250, which is also good. These numbers would indicate whether or not she would need a transfusion. Her counts have been that low before which is what results in the need for either a blood transfusion or a platelet transfusion. We are thankful that it doesn't appear she will need that right now, but know that it may be likely as she continues treatment and has to go through some more intense periods of chemotherapy. It's a good thing that she is 3 years old and that she could care less about what her bloodwork tells her the counts are....she is full of energy! She is happy and running around and getting lots of exercise. She is good about wearing her sunscreen on her head so it doesn't get burned, but Rob and I think she is going to probably be the tannest kid at clinic! It's hard to keep her inside...that's not a bad thing though.

She is excited about Easter, and we will be making a weekend trip down to Grandma and Grandpa's house while Daddy is on shift. With Grandma and Grandpa relocating to Tallahassee, there won't be many chances to head to Sarasota for holidays anymore, so this will be a good opportunity to spend time with family and friends. Taylor is also excited about going to the little white church.

I did get some additional info about the upcoming benefit on April 21st. Tickets will be available on Monday, April 9th for the event. Scheduled to appear is Swing Pocket (jazz, blues, and swing), Allie and the Allie Cats (rock / country), and Jason Byrd (country). Tickets are $10, and the proceeds are benefitting both the Burn Camp fundraiser as well as Taylor. For additional information, you can check out the Tallahassee Firefighters' website at http://www.iafflocal2339.org/. We hope to see you there!

Well, I will sign off for now as we will be headed out shortly for our trip. Love to all, and Happy Easter.

Love, Rob, Kim, Taylor and Alex

April 7, 2007

It is much chillier in south Florida than it should be! That didn't stop us from trying to head out to the beach to run around though- although when we got there...even Taylor said 'Mommy, it's too chilly!' We ended up staying for all of 5 minutes before loading back up into the car and heading for the house. Regardless, we continued to look for outside things to do while visiting Grandma and Grandpa, including a walk down to the lake near their house to see the turtles and the ducks.

We are trying to be a little more conservative about her activities, considering that her white blood cell count is down to 2.0. She seems to be feeling fine, but we just want to be sensitive to her counts, especially until we see the doctors at clinic again in a week or so. Being more conservative will most likely mean minimizing / eliminating eating out at restaurants all together, and resuming our avoidance of stores where there may be crowds of people. There was plenty that we found to do at home and outside before, so there will be plenty to do now.

She had a good time coloring Easter eggs this evening (and that was a good activity for keeping her awake to take her 6-MP before bedtime too). She is very excited about the Easter bunny coming tonight, and asked me several times if he would wait until she was asleep, or would he come when she was still awake. She is sleeping now, so I'm sure he will stop by shortly.

Well, I will try to get a picture of her and her little sister in their pretty Easter dresses tomorrow. Love to all, and Happy Easter!

Love, Rob, Kim, Taylor and Alex

April 8, 2007

We are back home in Tallahassee, and had a wonderful Easter weekend. Today was busy with sifting through treats from the Easter Bunny, going to Easter service, looking for eggs at the Easter egg hunt, and having dinner at Grandma and

Grandpa's house. Taylor also had the chance to visit some of the firefighters at Station #11 in Sarasota. Sarasota County firefighters, along with so many others across the state have been amazing to Taylor as she progresses through her treatments. We can't thank you guys enough.

We hope everyone had a wonderful Easter. The girls had a great day, and I tried to take pictures throughout the day...we've posted a few to the site. As you will see, it is tough to get a 3-year-old and a 16-month-old to pose for you at the same time!

I remember reading in a book recently that when a loved one is diagnosed with cancer or other life-threatening illnesses, holidays can feel bittersweet- meaning that they are happy times, but in the back of your mind...you wonder if this is the last one you will spend with them. I will admit the thought passed through my mind briefly at one point while she and I were dying Easter eggs last night; however, I did not see the point in dwelling on it. Besides the fact that we are focused on a positive outcome, and that there will be many more Easters to come, I try to remember that I don't know what tomorrow will bring...so I will be thankful for what we have today. And today was amazing.

Thank you for all of your good wishes and support. It was great to see our Sarasota church family and friends today, and thank you to Miss Genevieve and Dr. Jonathan for playing 'God Bless America' so Taylor could sing it after church! And thank you to Pastor Karl for Taylor's special trip to the little white church. She was very happy to get to visit.

Love to all, and we will continue to post about her progress this week.

Love, Rob, Kim, Taylor, and Alex

April 10, 2007

As I write this, Taylor is practicing her 'Dancing With the Stars' moves in her Cinderella gown. I will have to pull the video camera out one of these weeks, as she is always asking Daddy (a.k.a. Prince Charming) to dance with her. It is adorable. Grandma (our judge) has given her "10's" on all of her dances.

She is having a good week so far- still lots of energy, and a good appetite, so we are very happy. I spoke with one of her nurses today in Gainesville to make sure that we had calculated her ANC correctly last week. She confirmed the calculations we did last week based on the blood counts we received from KidsCorner, and explained that the drop from 1600+ to 780 shouldn't concern us. She said they expect the ANC to vary during this stage, and that she is still above 500, so she is not considered neutropenic right now. With her white blood cell count at 2.0 though, we are still being more conservative about her activities. We considered doing school pictures today, but passed...just in case someone may have had a runny nose! There will be many more class pictures to come, so missing this one will be okay.

I am looking forward to heading to Gainesville next week for her clinic visit and her procedure. There is a comfort level about the doctors and nurses seeing her in person and giving us feedback in person. I won't complain about not having to make the drive last week, and I'm sure that will be a nice option in the future too! But there is just that comfort level you get when talking to her doctors directly. They really are an amazing team. I have them to thank for every day we've had with her since January.

She is in good spirits, and had a good day playing with her friend Cole today. She is looking forward to the 'Relay for Life' this weekend, and is so excited about being a line leader as part of the survivor lap.

Love to all, and we'll keep you posted as the week goes on!

Love, Rob, Kim, Taylor, and Alex

April 12, 2007

Taylor had a good day with Alex and Daddy, and Mommy will be home with her and Alex tomorrow. She is getting ready for the 'Relay for Life' tomorrow night, and she had her Daddy load her wagon, her scooter, and a bike in the pickup truck tonight. She wants to be ready to go! I tried explaining to her tonight that she will get a special 'Survivor' t-shirt tomorrow night to wear. She didn't quite understand what the word 'survivor' meant, so I explained to her that it meant she gets to be a line leader around the track tomorrow night. She likes being the line leader, so she was happy. I'm sure tomorrow night will be filled with lots of emotions, but we just continue to be so proud of her.

Her daddy continues to amaze me with everything he is able to get done during the day. He sets the bar pretty high! He was able to move a bedroom set of furniture today downstairs (where our living room furniture used to be), and get Grandma's bedroom ready. Now she will have at least a little more of her own space while she is staying with us. He also managed to get the living room furniture moved to storage with the help of one of our friends (Thanks Doane!)....and get the girls fed and naps, etc. He is a great daddy and a great husband. I couldn't imagine going through all of this without him.

Taylor stopped by my office today for a visit, and she was happy to come inside for a few minutes. Her favorite thing to do is get a snack from the vending machine, and then draw on my white board. She got a little shy when she walked in, but then warmed up a bit and even said Hi to some folks there.

We'll take lots of pictures at the Relay, and get them posted. She will head to Gainesville next week, and we will get a sense of how she is progressing in her current phase. As we get closer to mid-May and the 'delayed intensification' phase, I will admit, I start to get pretty stressed. I know it will be a tough time on her little body and mind, and it will be a time for Rob and I to lean on each other that much more. I won't worry about that today though. Today was a very good day, so I'll focus on that.

Love to all...Rob, Kim, Taylor and Alex

April 15, 2007

Wow...what a weekend. We kicked off this weekend with the Relay for Life on Friday night / Saturday morning. I cannot even explain what an emotional experience it was. Leading up to the Relay, I don't think it fully hit me that it would be a night of tears and roller coaster emotions, but what a wonderful experience. And, what a wonderful honor. Taylor was the honored child survivor for this event, and had the opportunity to help lead the survivor lap. While she had brought a scooter, a wagon, a bike and a stroller, she opted for Mommy to carry her for that line leader lap. I think it was all a little overwhelming for her at first, but after a lap or two- we had to keep up with her! She rode her bike and her scooter around the track, took laps in her wagon, including a lap with her good friend Dawson...and then there were just the laps where she ran!

As part of the event, Taylor and I also had the chance to say a few words during the opening event. As we were about to go on stage, that is when the tears first came over me...She was just standing there talking to her friends (Abbie and Camryn...who she wanted to come on stage with her) and I was just watching her. What hit me all at once was that she was wearing a purple t-shirt that 'Survivor' on it, and my mind started spinning and thinking: "She's only 3 years old- how did we get here? How is it that our child is 3 and can already be a survivor of anything? She hasn't been around that long to need to have experienced this..." Several thoughts like that started going through my mind, and I turned around so that the crowd and Taylor wouldn't see my crying...but Taylor saw. She came over to me and said "What's wrong Mommy?" and I told a fib and said "Oh, Mommy was just yawning real big, and my eyes started to water..." and then she touched my face with both of her hands and said "Why does your face look like that then?" and I told her, "I don't know, but can you help make it happy again?" and so she did...she started tickling my face and laughing, and we were ready to go on stage.

I can't thank all of the Relay participants enough, and of course I was so honored that there were 2 teams out there walking for Taylor: 'Team Princess Taylor' and 'Team Taylor and Niki.' You guys were all so amazing...pulling the all-nighter and raising an amazing amount of money for research. I had some great conversations with friends and co-workers as we did those laps around the track the other night (and when we took some breaks at the tent too!) Many thanks to Lori, Alana and Joy for their team captain roles in coordinating the respective teams. The support that we've received from all of you, including the time you've taken to support this event means so much. Rob and I are forever appreciative.

Alex had a good time at the Relay as well, and had a chance to play with lots of friends, including little Charlie from Atlanta. He and his Mommy drove down to participate in the event as part of 'Team Princess Taylor,' and we were so happy to see them. Aunt Kim and Mommy go back to college days, so this weekend was a great opportunity to get caught up on everything that's been going on over the past 3 months. I miss those late-night talks!!!

The rest of the weekend was spent getting some catch up sleep and getting Taylor's room ready with her new bunk beds. Taylor's previous furniture is now down in Grandma's bedroom (a.k.a. our old living room), and the bunk beds are a great fit in Taylor's room. She is constantly watching for Alex to make sure she isn't climbing up the ladder. They take good care of each other.

We had a little bit of a scare with what we think is a challenge with Taylor's sugar level this morning. She woke up cold, clammy, lethargic, and nauseated. After some Gatorade, she did get sick, but then was able to eat. Within 15 minutes of eating, she had her energy level back, and maintained that the remainder of the day. She never did have a temperature, but this is something we want the doctors to give us some more advice about when we see them this week.

Well, I am headed upstairs to bed, but wanted to send our love to all. We hope to see you at the benefit this coming Saturday (April 21st). Rob and I have tickets if you want to call us directly or please visit http://www.iafflocal2339.org/benefit.htm for additional info.

We'll keep you posted as the week progresses!

April 19, 2007

Getting ready to head to Gainesville today. Taylor will go to clinic today to see the doctors and to get labs drawn so that they can assess her blood counts. They will access her port as well, and then leave her accessed for a procedure that she will have tomorrow. Tomorrow's procedure will be the first LP (lumbar puncture) that she has had to have in over a month, so it has been a nice break. Typically, she handles the procedures well, and recovers quickly, so we are anticipating a return trip home tomorrow from Gainesville. Today is her Daddy's birthday, so I think it is a little ironic that he will spend it in Gainesville, but he reminded me that it is the best birthday present in the world if his little girl continues to get better. I think so too.

She packed her own suitcase last night, and she seriously packed for a week! I explained that she was only going for 1 night, but she said she didn't know if it would be hot or cold when she woke up the next morning (hence the shorts, sweatpants, sweaters, and short sleeve shirts). I guess it is good that she is so prepared! It all fit in one suitcase, so what's the difference if she brought 1 night's clothes? Or a week's worth?

Last night, she headed out to a 'King of the Hill' softball game sponsored by the firefighters. It's a game where the legislators play for fun (Republicans vs. Democrats)She had a really good time last night, and got to see lots of the firefighters who have been praying and supporting for her through all of this. It started to get chilly though, so Mommy and Taylor headed home for bath time, medicine time, and bedtime.

She continues to be our brave little girl, and has been having a lot of energy. We know she will be excited to go to the benefit this Saturday night. We'll confirm with the doctors that her counts are good enough, and that it will be okay for her to go...but we are very hopeful that it won't be an issue. Rob and I have tickets, so please contact us directly if you are interested....or you can check out the website (http://www.iafflocal2339.org/) for additional info. It is this Saturday night at 8 p.m. at the American Legion Hall. We hope to see you there!

Love to all, and we will keep you posted about her trip to clinic today. Thank you again for everything- your prayers and support are surrounding her and helping her every day.

Love, Rob, Kim, Taylor and Alex

April 19, 2007

Taylor had a great day at clinic! Her ANC was 975 (up from 780 two weeks ago), so that was very good news. Part of this calculation is her white blood cell count, which was up from 2.0 to 2.5 this week. Additionally, her hematocrit was 34, her hemoglobin was 12, and her platelets were 155. These levels were good, so there was no need to consider any transfusions prior to her procedure tomorrow. We were happy about that! Rob said that she did great when the nurses accessed her port (a.k.a., her 'buddy'), and that Taylor continued to help them with getting the blood in the vacutainers for her labs. They also ran a complete metabolic panel (a CMP is what I believe Rob called it for short). This was done to help assess any issues with her sugar. Rob received a call back from the doctors this evening, and it indicated that her glucose was 117. While this was a little high for a child (they said that the upper end of the range for kids would be 100), the doctors did not see a reason to be concerned at this point. They also went back and reviewed each of her CMPs that were done previously, and her glucose levels were all within the normal range. Taylor had just eaten prior to the CMP today, so this could have also been a factor. They asked us to just keep an eye on her to see if this is a continuing issue, and I feel confident that they will help us work through any questions about it. Overall, the doctors are happy with her progress and energy levels, so it was a great day.

She starts a 5-day steroid regimen tomorrow, and will continue with her other medicines (6-MP, Methotrexate, and Septra). While the times on steroids can be tough, the 5-day stints are much better than the 29-day stint during Induction. Rob and I are considering getting her the 'Decadron' pills instead of the liquid that we've given her before. She is doing so well taking her other pills, so we figure getting Decadron in a pill form will make medicine time less difficult.

Today was time well spent with Alex too. Even though Alex is so young, I know she must miss 'her normal routine' of getting to go to Granny's house (her home daycare) and playing with her friends....so having a day of undivided attention from Mommy was nice. When the doctors tell us that Taylor is well enough to return to school (on a full or part time basis), then we will also assess if Alex should go back. Her exposure to other kids and germs is something we just have to be sensitive about.

With Taylor's counts being at an acceptable level, and assuming a successful return trip home after her procedure tomorrow, it looks like she will be able to attend the benefit this Saturday night! There is still time to get tickets, and you can contact Rob or I directly if you need them. I have some on hand, and am more than happy to get them to you tomorrow or Saturday. For more info about the event, you can also check out the website at http://www.iafflocal2339.org/.

Look forward to seeing folks on Saturday night, and thank you again for all of your prayers and support.

Love, Rob, Kim, Taylor, and Alex

April 23, 2007

Another amazing weekend...and a busy one too; hence, the lack of journal updates until today!

Taylor's LP went well on Friday, with the exception of a tough time in the recovery room following the procedure. We have found that if Taylor wakes up in the recovery room, and either Mommy or Daddy aren't there...the nurses are in for quite a show (yelling, screaming, crying). I can't blame her though. She's only 3, and scared to death. For that reason, the nurses typically come and get either Rob or I prior to her waking up from the procedure. That way, when she wakes up...she sees one of us, and isn't scared. Unfortunately, timing on Friday must have been off. Rob didn't receive word to go back to the recovery room until it was too late. That resulted in an extra 2 hours at Shands with Rob trying to calm Taylor down and get her into her car seat for the trip home. As frustrating as that was, the good news is that she did come home on Friday, so we eventually put that into perspective.

Friday continued to be a good day, with family coming into town for Taylor's benefit on Saturday night. Aunt Kathy and Gammy arrived on Friday, and got to spend lots of time with the girls. Taylor and Aunt Kathy also went with Alex and me for Alex's first haircut. What a big day for Alex! Alex did great though. She climbed right up in the chair- no need to even sit on Mommy's lap. What a big girl! When we were at the salon, Taylor decided she needed her bangs trimmed up too. Times like that are so sweet- you don't know whether to laugh or cry!

Friday was also fun because Miss Ally came by to visit with Taylor. Taylor had a good time showing her the princess room and doing puzzles. Saturday was time well spent with family, including Uncle Jack, Aunt Gwen, Luke and Miss Sharon who came to town for the benefit. We cooked out and spent lots of time outside playing with everyone in the neighborhood on Saturday afternoon which was nice for the kids. Then it was time to get ready for the party...Taylor was adorable. She wore a pretty green dress and her black shoes, and took lots of time getting ready. At one point, I was downstairs saying "Taylor, it's time to go," and she said "Hold on Mommy, I am putting on some makeup so I can look the beautifullest." I went upstairs, and there she was- standing on the stool in her bathroom trying to put on eyeshadow and blush. I told her that even without the makeup, she was still the beautifullest...and we were on our way. Because the party didn't start until 8 p.m., little sister Alex stayed home. With bedtime at 8 p.m., she would not have enjoyed the party. There will be plenty of pictures though!

The benefit was great. Thank you to everyone who came out. Your love and support has been so appreciated! Taylor danced the night away. She was so happy to see some of her friends too. Madison and Abbie were there, and then of course, she loved having cousin Luke there! The kids were a hit, and danced nonstop for each of the bands on stage. Watching them made the rest of us tired! But it also reminded me of how blessed we are that she continues to have the energy level she does. And she was just having so much fun. Rob and I can't thank the firefighters enough for including Taylor as part of the benefit. From the moment Taylor received her diagnosis, they have just been amazing. It is a support network I would wish on everyone.

The weekend continued with a 'Family Fun Day' out at Little River farm. Thank you so much to the Knox family for having us out yesterday. It was just such a nice opportunity for families to get together at the farm for a cook out and to play. There was fishing, riding around the farm on jeeps and four wheelers, a bounce house, and my

favorite- some nice rocking chairs on the porch for just sitting and relaxing! Taylor and Alex had a great time with their friends, and played really hard (which made bedtime pretty smooth last night too). Mr. Craig helped Taylor catch a fish, which she was very excited about, and she loved riding on the four-wheeler with her Daddy. Like I said earlier, we continue to feel blessed with her energy level right now. It allows her to continue to experience so many fun things, and for life to be as normal as it can be.

I've posted some pictures from this weekend, and then will be posting pictures from the benefit when I receive copies this week (With everything going on, I left the camera at home on Saturday night...but folks are sending me their pictures!) Thanks to everyone who took pictures on Saturday evening. Taylor had an amazing time.

Love to all, and we will keep you posted on her week. We are checking in with the doctors today to understand when her next blood count check will be, as she does not need to go back to Gainesville for a formal visit until next month. Our assumption is that she will need to go for a 2 week check here at KidsCorner, but we'll check with them today. Take care!

Love, Rob, Kim, Taylor, and Alex

April 26, 2007

Taylor's week has continued to go well. We are constantly amazed at her energy level, and we remember to be thankful for it every day. We checked in with her doctors, and she will need to go for a visit next week to get her blood drawn, but that can be done locally. So, assuming no other issues arise, we shouldn't have to go to Gainesville for a visit until mid-May. At that point, she will begin the 'delayed intensification' phase, and I believe that visits will become more frequent again....but that's okay!

We had a slight scare earlier in the week when we found out

that she had possibly been exposed to strep throat this past weekend. The concern would be her suppressed immunity at the moment (due to the chemotherapy regimen), so it is something that could have been concerning. We called her doctors as soon as we found out, and they said to just keep an eye on her for symptoms. We also proactively called our doctors to see if Rob or I should take any additional precautions (i.e., get a prescription so that we helped her avoid any other exposure). To date, no symptoms have showed up, so we are counting our blessings there as well.

She has had a great week, even with the dose of steroids she was on. The effects seemed less than last month, but she still was a little 'hypersensitive' about a lot of things. Overall though, she continues to amaze us. She has enjoyed playing with friends, going on walks, and helping Mommy and Daddy cook too. She made special dessert last night to surprise Daddy (chocolate and vanilla pudding mixed together). She was very excited about that.

Well, love to all, and we will keep you posted on her progress!

Love, Rob, Kim, Taylor and Alex

April 27, 2007

I should know better than to jinx us with saying that she hasn't shown up with symptoms!!! This morning, Taylor woke up with a scratchy throat, runny nose and upset tummy. We are working with her doctors and keeping an eye on her to see how she works through this, and to see if any further action is needed, but for now, we just have to wait and see. That is definitely the tough part, as you feel very out of control! I think Dax (one of Taylor's nurses at Shands) could sense that in my voice this morning. He told me 'I know you're worried,' and I told him that the waiting part is just tough. I'm sure he has had to help advise several families on stuff like this, and I know that Shands will work with us to get her what she needs.

Her energy level remains high and she is in good spirits, so we will keep an eye on her as this works its way through her system. Thank you to everyone for your continued prayers. They help her every day!

Love, Rob, Kim, Taylor and Alex

April 30, 2007

I had already updated the journal for today, but then Rob read me Carson's website (Taylor's friend from school: www. caringbridge.org/visit/carsonchapman). Carson is back at Shands after some tough episodes this week, most recently a seizure this weekend. From his website update, it also appears that he needed additional transfusions. I know how scared his parents are feeling right now. This is part of the unknown that we are living with every day, and you just want it all to be better. While we are happy that Taylor continues to fight off her cold germs from this week, it reminds us of the vulnerable state that she is in right now. Carson is in good hands though, and we pray that he will be home soon.

Taylor's cold seems to be doing okay, and she spent the weekend playing with Grandma and Grandpa and helping them look for a new house. She has her own set of criteria when she helps them look- her primary one being whether or not the house already has a swing set in the backyard. Those tend to be her favorite....Overall, her energy level and spirits remain high, which is what always gives us comfort.

She continues to take her medicine, and wants to be so independent. If she could open the child proof caps on her own, she wouldn't want Rob or I to even help! Rob and I were talking about how much of her 'independence' is coming back to her. When all of this started, there was definitely (and understandably) a regression. She wouldn't dress herself, go to the bathroom without assistance, etc. Now, she'll come downstairs in the morning fully dressed, teeth brushed and room cleaned. My favorite was last night though. After dinner, she ran upstairs for bath time. By the time I got upstairs, she was already running the bathwater, had put her clothes in the hamper, and had Alex helping her get washcloths. She said she wanted to surprise us. Since she and Alex have to take separate baths, Taylor takes a bath in Rob's and my bathroom for now (which has a garden tub). Last night, she went on to explain to me that she would like to take a relaxing bath with music and a drink to sip (i.e., her Gatorade juice box). I had to put a stop if it had come to candles too...I mean, she is only 3! It was adorable though. I guess you just have to cherish silly moments like that in the midst of all of the craziness that goes on.

As we get closer to mid-May and delayed intensification, I do get a little nervous; however, I don't want it to be a self-fulfilling prophecy! I do think there will be some things that will be 'easier' (if you can imagine!) as compared to the initial 'Induction' period. My dad and I were talking about this over the weekend....For example- taking medicine multiple times per day is just part of Taylor's routine now. That was something totally new to her 3 months ago (and the time(s) of day we dreaded the most). Additionally, her ability to take pills as opposed to liquid has made the whole process a lot smoother. We'll be able to benefit from that to the extent possible in this next phase too. Rob and I are also prepared for the physical changes that will be coming, and might be able to help Taylor understand them a little better this time too. She understands that the medicine does funny things, including making our tummy bigger, making us want to eat all of the time, etc. We expect that we'll see some of those same side effects as part of this phase. There will be some new medicines though, and we may have to better understand those effects, but I also remind myself that we are talking about a 2-month period before getting back to the chemo regimen she's on now. We can get through this!

All we can do is be thankful for her progress to date and the happy days we have been having. I pray that these cold germs will continue to go away, and that her counts are acceptable this week when she has her labs drawn. We will keep you posted, and are always so appreciative of everyone's love and support.

Love, Rob, Kim, Taylor, and Alex

April 30, 2007

I had the chance to talk to Carson's mom today. It was good to hear her voice and hear that Carson has been doing okay since he has been down at Shands. Like I said this morning, I know Carson is in good hands (with the doctors and his family), and talking to his mom today just reminded me what a strong woman she is and is having to be right now... We will continue to pray that his stay at Shands is short, and that he'll be home quickly.

Taylor's energy level continued to remain high today; however, both her daddy and I noticed that she started to look a little pale. While we were going to wait until Thursday to take her for her lab work, we are now going to try to get in for her blood draw tomorrow. Her runny nose continued, and I guess it will just take her body a little longer to fight it off (than it would have 6 months ago), but something seemed to cause her to look a little more drained today. Having said that, she still felt good enough tonight to get dressed in her ball gown for 'Dancing with the Stars.' Sadly, I had forgotten it was Monday night (i.e., one of our 'Dancing with the Stars' nights), but I was quickly reminded of that at dinner. I let Alex stay up for the first dance, and Taylor tried to teach her how to waltz, and it ended up more like a wrestling match. It was adorable.

We will keep you posted on whether we are able to get her labs drawn tomorrow and what the results are. Thank you for your continued thoughts and prayers.

Love, Rob, Kim, Taylor, and Alex

May 1, 2007

Today was a long day, and one that felt like an emotional rollercoaster. I am glad that Rob and I trusted our gut yesterday about needing to get her counts checked. Taylor, Alex and I headed to KidsCorner today (the lab here locally at Tallahassee Memorial). When I say Taylor is one of the bravest people I know, I am in constant admiration of her. She decided she wanted to bring her scooter to the hospital today, and she rode it into the hospital and up to KidsCorner (mask on and all). She also continued to demonstrate her amazing attitude when she had her 'buddy' accessed to get her labs drawn. When the results came back, her ANC came back at 117. This was concerning, as her last ANC was 975 (less than 2 weeks ago). Being under 500 also means that she is neutropenic, and extremely susceptible to infection. We checked her labs from the past 3 months, and her counts haven't been this low since February 2nd. It was like rewinding to being back in Gainesville prior to coming back to Tallahassee. The great news is that her hemoglobin was 10, her hematocrit was 30 and her platelets were 200. These were all at a level where the doctors are not needing to consider a transfusion. Additionally, her energy level has been great today, but with an ANC of 112, there is enough reason for concern that her doctors at Shands are having us stop her chemo meds (6-MP and Methotrexate) for the next week.

When Rob called me with the news about stopping the chemo meds, I pretty much lost it. I can't totally explain why. Maybe I was afraid that being off of the chemo- even for a week- would risk her progress in some way. But I guess I wanted to be mad at something, or blame someone or something, and bless my husband who just let me yell and vent. So I started yelling and asking 'What is happening?' 'What did she catch?' 'Why can't she just get an antibiotic and get rid of this cold? That has to be the reason this is happening...it's not the medicine...' I was pretty much all over the place. But then again, when I came to the realization that I don't have an 'MD' after my name, Rob also conveyed additional explanations from the doctors to me. He explained that her chemo medications are continuing to kill bad cells and good cells. Because her good cells may be down, she is just that much more susceptible to germs. It means we have to resume being extremely cautious again. This means that we will also become extremely protective again about exposure to other kids, having people over to the house, etc. The doctors explained that if her temperature gets to 100.4 degrees, we will need to have her admitted to the hospital for a minimum of 48 hours so she can have IV antibiotics. During that 48-hour timeframe, they will also try to grow cultures of whatever would be causing the fever. I would prefer not to even have to do this though.

Upon returning home today, the cloroxing and cleaning began. Even though it feels like we are constantly cleaning, it went to the next level today. When I tell you I was using a toothbrush with bleach on the bathrooms today, I'm not kidding. If there is a germ in this house, it better get out of my way.

To put it in perspective, I think today was the most scared we've felt since her diagnosis. For the most part, I feel like we've settled into our routine- we got over the initial shock of the diagnosis, we do daily medicines, we make our trips to Gainesville, we keep our notebook with extensive information about every visit and lab draw she has had, and we get through each day being thankful that we've had another day with Taylor. And I would say that lately, I have taken for granted that she has been making it through this phase with minimal to no issues. And then you have a day like today. I held her so tight tonight when I put her to bed. She fell asleep downstairs waiting for 'Dancing with the Stars' to begin. I carried her up the stairs and just rocked her for a few minutes and sang her a lullaby before tucking her into her Princess bed. Then I just took time to watch her sleep and say a little prayer before leaving her room. I asked God to please let her get past this episode and any episodes that may happen during treatment. I asked him to please let her stay with us, and that I don't want her leaving us to be part of his plan. I'll remember to pray for more strength tonight.

I am telling myself this is just a bump in the road, but it brings us back to the reality that this is a marathon, not a sprint...Thank you for your prayers. I know they are helping her stay strong...We will keep you posted, as she will be having subsequent checks within the week for her blood counts.

Love, Rob, Kim, Taylor and Alex

May 4, 2007

Taylor had a great day. She and Alex spent lots of time with Daddy, and went to the park for a picnic too. She is continuing to fight off her cold germs, and her energy level has been great. When I got home from work tonight, we spent some time playing outside and she showed Grandpa how she drives Alex around in the Barbie jeep.

We've had a couple of days to settle into not taking medicine at night, and at the end of the day- everything is just fine. I have come to the understanding that this is just going to be part of the treatment...there will be times where her regimen will need to be adjusted. It has helped that so many of you have reached out to help explain that to me too, so thank you. Your words of encouragement and examples of how you or your loved ones have gone through this were reassuring.

I was talking to a friend tonight about a book I was reading. The book mentioned that although the phrase 'God won't give you more than you can handle' is a common phrase....it is nowhere to be found in the Bible. I've used that phrase many times myself. Since Taylor's diagnosis, I think I've realized that God may give you more than you can handle, but he

97

also gives you a support network to get through it. Rob and I are so thankful for the support of family and friends, as this has helped us get through this time. Many thanks to Grandma and Grandpa who are keeping an eye on the kids so that Rob and I can get away this weekend for our 5th anniversary. We won't be too far away, but as several folks have reminded us- it is important for he and I to make time for each other too. I guess it's all part of getting things back to normal...Taylor and Alex will be in good hands, and we will be a phone call away.

We will keep you posted on her progress. She will have her counts checked again on Tuesday, and we are hopeful for them to have gone up. Take care.

Love, Rob, Kim, Taylor and Alex

May 7, 2007

Taylor had a great weekend, and continues to fight off those cold germs! She had a great time with Grandma, Grandpa, and Aunt Debbie, and is continuing to keep her energy levels up. We are trying to make sure that she eats a reasonable balance of foods, but thankfully she is eating a sufficient amount of protein. Her typical breakfast is 4-5 slices of turkey and some cheese, so she is starting her day off with good energy. We keep telling her that the protein will help her build big muscles and to stay strong. She is drinking plenty of fluids too, so we are hopeful that her cold will soon be completely gone.

We have an appointment with KidsCorner tomorrow morning to have her counts checked again. Following the appointment and receiving her results, we'll check in with her doctors to understand if it is okay to resume her chemo medications. If so, she'll start back with her 6-MP tomorrow night.

Today is a beautiful day in Tallahassee...in the mid-high 70's and breezy. It has been a nice day for the kids to play outside, and Taylor has been riding her bike. She even took her bike with her when she made a trip to see Granny today. Alex and Taylor gave Granny hugs and kisses, and played outside in the driveway for a good hour or so.

Well, the girls are napping now, but should be up shortly. We're headed back outside to keep exercising those legs...We'll let everyone know how her lab work comes back. Thank you again for all of your nice postings and encouraging words.

Love, Rob, Kim, Taylor, and Alex

May 9, 2007

Taylor went to KidsCorner yesterday, and her counts are up to 391. While it is good news that they are up, they are still not high enough to resume her chemotherapy medications. Her counts need to be at least 750, so her doctors would like us to hold off on her medication for another week. One additional change is that they will have us hold off on her Septra (her antibiotic) too. Her doctors explained that the Septra can sometimes be 'count suppressive,' so holding off on this may also help her counts to come back up. The great news is that her hemoglobin was up to 11.7 her hematocrit was up to 33.5, and her platelets were 306. All of these were in the normal range which is very reassuring.

We are supposed to talk to her doctors again today to understand the impact (i.e., potential delay) that this could have on her moving into the next phase (delayed intensification). In reading the literature that they have provided us, it doesn't appear that holding off on the medicine along should delay it, but we want to just clarify that. Instead, our current understanding is that her ANC has to be at 750 and her platelets have to be at 75 in order to move to the next phase.

We pray that her counts will continue to come up, and that her hematocrit, hemoglobin, and platelets stay high as well. We are just taking each day one at a time, and will be in Gainesville next week.

Thank you for your love and support. She will most likely have her counts checked within the week again, so we will keep you posted.

Love, Rob, Kim, Taylor and Alex

May 10, 2007

We had a chance to verify some information with Taylor's doctors today. The goal is for her counts to be at 750 and 75 by next Thursday. That means that her ANC needs to be at 750 (the calculation that considers her white blood cells and her neutrophils), and her platelets need to be at 75. With the current phase that she is in, the roadmap does not require that she make up any time lost with the 6-MP and oral Methotrexate from the past 2 weeks. Because those are the only medications she has missed, there is not a reason to delay going to the next phase (assuming that her counts are acceptable). That was good news to hear as we want her to continue through her treatment; however, we also understand that her body needs to be healthy enough to handle the treatment. Her doctors didn't see a need to have her counts checked again prior to next Thursday when we are in Gainesville, so we will wait until then. At that point, we'll know whether her counts are high enough to begin 'delayed intensification' that day (including an overnight stay for an LP on Friday morning). We'll pack our suitcases with the hope that we will be having the LP on Friday morning, but we'll have a better sense when we get to clinic on Thursday. If it is meant to be that next week is the right time for her to begin the next phase of treatment, it will be the right time. If it's not, it just means that her body needs more time to build back up. I think I'm coming to a better understanding about all of that.

We'll keep everyone posted, and thank you again for your prayers for Taylor. I received some pictures tonight of Taylor at the Firefighters' benefit in April, and have posted a couple on Taylor's site. Looking at them reminded me of how much fun she had that night. She literally danced non-stop (well, maybe a break or two! but that's it!). Thanks to Miss Jacquie for sending along....Take care.

Love, Rob, Kim, Taylor, and Alex

May 15, 2007

Taylor has had a great weekend. Aunt Peggy came to visit, and the kids have enjoyed spending time with her. Taylor and Alex (with some help from Daddy) took her for a picnic on a pontoon boat, they have spent time at the park, and Taylor has been helping her do some baking too! I was talking to a friend last night about how comforting it has been to have so much support- family, friends....everyone.

We are getting ready to make our next trip to Gainesville. It is a little bit of an anxious trip, as we will know (based on her counts on Thursday) whether she will move on to the next phase of 'delayed intensification.' Rob and I have been reviewing the roadmap for this next phase, and it will definitely be different from the most recent phase of 'Standard Interim Maintenance.' There are new drug therapies, more intense chemo, as well as more frequent trips to Shands, but that is okay as this is all part of the plan for Taylor to get better. There will be things to prepare her for again, such as the shots of 'PEG' that she will need to receive- the first of which will be next week (most likely Monday, Tuesday or Wednesday of next week). The 'PEG' shot is given in her leg, and the last time she had one of those was Day 4 of her Induction phase. The advice from the counselors at Shands is to prepare her for things like this, but because of her age, the suggestion is to tell her that day. That makes sense or else her poor little mind will be scared thinking about it. So- lots for us to think about in the coming weeks. I pray that her little body will continue to stay strong and fight through the side effects of these medicines.

Overall, her energy level remains good and she is in great spirits. She watched 'Dancing with the Stars' last night with

Grandma and Aunt Peggy, and she is hopeful that Joey will make it to the next round. Writing about that reminded me that I wanted to pass along another amazing thing that Shands does. They work with a foundation called 'Dreams Come True' to help children with life threatening illnesses experience a wish. They have ways of asking questions directly of the children so that they can find a 'true' wish for the child- which I think is just amazing. They talked to Taylor during her last visit to clinic about what her wish would be, and she told them that she would like to go see 'Dancing With the Stars.' Their team is working to see if they can make this wish come true. If so, it may be something down the line (as she wouldn't be able to make that trip now), but I was so excited for her that she had a wish so unique to her. It is hard to come to a realization that your child has a 'life threatening' illness, but she does, and just like them- I want to make sure she has lots of happy experiences. I am so happy that foundations such as this exist, and do the amazing things they do for children.

We will keep everyone posted on the outcome of her trip to Gainesville this week. Thank you again for your prayers and support. As we enter this next phase, I feel that Rob and I will continue to find strength we did not even know we had, but we know that God is giving us a network of support to help us find that strength. Take care.

Love, Rob, Kim, Taylor, and Alex

May 18, 2007

And we are back from Gainesville....

The past 2 days have been long, but good. Taylor started with a trip to clinic yesterday where she had her counts done, had an echocardiogram (an ultrasound of her heart), and had 2 chemo drugs via her 'buddy' (which signified the kickoff for the next round of chemotherapy....delayed intensification).

The doctors needed to do the echocardiogram to get a baseline of her heart function (prior to administering some of the new drugs during the 'delayed intensification' phase of treatment). While the fact that heart issues could even be a concern is kind of scary, I appreciate that Taylor's doctors are extremely cautious and are making sure that she is okay through all of this. She did great having her 'buddy' accessed when Nurse Amy drew blood for her counts, and was so excited to get to help with flushing her buddy and getting the blood in the vacutainers for the lab. An interesting point is that Taylor's ANC was 625, which we would have thought would have had the doctors hold off on moving to delayed intensification; however, they reminded me that those are guidelines, and that judgement calls are used throughout the course of treatment...makes sense to me! Additionally, in looking at some other factors from her blood (specifically her monocytes and her neutrophils), the doctors felt good about her moving forward. I trust her team of doctors, and I know that they do this a lot more than I do, so she began her next round as of yesterday. I also reminded myself of something I said just the other day on the website about having to turn this over to God and trust that he is giving the doctors the knowledge and tools to make Taylor better. With regard to other key points from her labs...her hemoglobin was 12.5, her hematocrit was 34.6, and her platelets were 191. These were all within a normal range which is comforting (and not near levels requiring a transfusion). Her white blood cell count was 2.5, which continues to be low, but acceptable enough to move forward.

The 2 chemo drugs that Taylor had at clinic yesterday were Vincristine and Doxorubicin. Taylor has had Vincristine throughout her treatment to date; however, yesterday was the first-time having Doxorubicin. The Doxorubicin is the drug that triggered the need for the echocardiogram, so I am hopeful that it is doing its job without having any bad side effects. One interesting side effect (and one that Taylor was quite excited about) is that it makes her urine red. She was thrilled to hear this, and ran to the potty at least twice at clinic (right after they administered it) to see if she was 'peeing red' yet. The red tint didn't kick in until we got to the hotel, but boy was she excited. I whispered a little prayer of thanks to God that he has helped by throwing in humorous situations in the midst of all of this!

This morning, she had a lumbar puncture (LP) at the hospital where they administered intrathecal Methotrexate (putting the Methotrexate in her spine). She was a brave little girl, and even came out of recovery just fine this time around. In fact, she was pretty loopy from the 'sleepy juice' that they gave her. She kept on telling me she was seeing 'two froggy tattoos' (although they had only given her one during the procedure). Eventually her double vision subsided, and she wanted some McDonald's for the trip home...Again, some humor in the midst of all of this I guess.

So- all in all, a good trip to Gainesville. We are back home tonight, and began her medicine regimen for this phase. I will ask that everyone pray for the ability for her to rest well, as her steroid dosage is quite high during this phase as compared to previous phases. Previously, she took 2.0 mg of her Decadron in the morning, and 1.5 mg in the evening. During this phase, she will take 3.25 of Decadron in the morning, and 3.0 mg in the evening. Her doctors reminded me of the word 'intense' in this phase (delayed intensification), and that this will include higher dosages of medicine than in previous phases. Needless to say, we expect the steroids to really kick in over the next few days, and with that to come some trying times....but it is a 21-day regimen, and we know that we can get through it. I guess we are 1 day down, 20 to go! This phase will bring with it additional new medicines, so we pray that her little body has minimal side effects from them.

Thank you again for all of your kind words and support. We will keep you posted as she heads back to Gainesville for visits on Tuesday and Thursday of next week. She is a strong-willed little girl, and as tough as this phase will be, I have no doubt that she will continue to prove that to us. Love to all...

Love, Rob, Kim, Taylor and Alex

May 21, 2007

Today was a good day overall. She had a fun day with Daddy and Alex, and had a chance to play with her friends in the neighborhood too. This evening was a little tougher though as Taylor started to get tired and get frustrated. You can start to see the effects of the steroids as she is struggling with her emotions and having outbursts from time to time. I think Rob and I have been better prepared this time, and are expecting the outbursts...so we are also ready to talk her through it and are trying to be as calm as possible with her. It is hard though, as you don't know what is going to trigger her emotions, but we are just trying our best, and we know she is not herself when the outbursts happen. Tonight her outbursts were triggered by the fact that (1) I was talking during 'The Wheel of Fortune' and (2) I was out of Saltine crackers. I'm sure this would be frustrating to most people, so what was I thinking???

Thankfully, the outbursts were short, and she eventually fell asleep. Sadly, she was not able to stay awake through 'Dancing with the Stars,' but I recorded it for her so that she can watch it tomorrow when we get back from Gainesville. I am going to vote on her behalf tonight for Joey. Hopefully her vote will help him in the final show tomorrow...we shall see!

Tomorrow she will get her PEG shots while we are at clinic. We will be able to use some of the 'numbing' cream on her legs, so that should help in easing some of the pain from the shots. I am sure that it will be hard to get her back in the car to go back to Gainesville on Thursday, but we'll deal with that then!

Well, I am headed to bed now so I can be ready in case she

wakes up at some point during the night. Her daddy has been amazing at taking care of her the past few nights when she wakes up, and letting me get some sleep. He is wonderful.

I will provide an update tomorrow night once we return from clinic. Thank you again for keeping up with her progress.

Love, Rob, Kim, Taylor, and Alex

May 23, 2007

Taylor did amazing yesterday at clinic. She was very brave when she got her PEG shot, even though she told me 'I wasn't brave Mommy because I cried a little bit.' I explained to her that sometimes even really brave people cry, and that she was the bravest little girl I knew! She is pretty smart too. Let me explain... Rob and I had discussed not telling her about the shot until right before they were about to give it. (At her age, it would serve no purpose for her to worry about it all the way to clinic. It would have been extremely stressful for her). However, thank you very much to Nurse Amy and Miss Shay (Carson's mommy) who suggested putting the 'numbing' cream on Taylor's legs before we got to clinic. When I put it on her legs, she asked me 'Mommy, are they going to put needles in my legs today?' She didn't seem scared, just really intrigued that they would have to do that at clinic. I didn't want to lie to her, but I also knew it was best not to upset her either, so I told her 'That's a good question. We'll need to ask them when we get to clinic.' So, she got her shot, and moved on. She was more interested in showing Alex the puzzles and books and games at clinic, and she even picked out a 'ring pop' for both her and Alex. It was a good day overall.

After clinic, we headed to Payne's Prairie state park for a visit. This was really special because some really nice folks at DEP (Department of Environmental Protection) had sent Taylor and Alex each a passport book. This book lists all of the state parks and there is a place for 'stamps' from each park. As soon as we got to the ranger station at the park, Taylor said 'Is this where we get the stamps Mommy?' She had a great time. It was a perfect day....a deer walked right in front of our car, we saw a turtle, and we saw a red bird. Taylor and Alex loved it.

Many thanks to Grandma who made the trip with us yesterday....it was a nice girls' trip. We will keep you posted on our clinic trip tomorrow. Love to all, and we will post an update tomorrow.

Love, Rob, Kim, Taylor, and Alex

May 24, 2007

The whole family made the trip to Gainesville today, and had a pleasant surprise when Taylor had her labs drawn. Her ANC was up over 4000! (4582 to be exact). When Rob and I looked at the lab sheet, our jaws hit the ground- after the new medicines she has been taking, we were hoping she would just be at least 500! Her doctors reminded us that the steroids help to keep her white blood cells boosted, which I guess was evident as her white blood cell count was 5.8. Her platelets were 178, her hemoglobin was 14.1, and her hematocrit was 40.4. These are all high enough to not worry about a transfusion at the moment, so we were happy. We have heard that transfusions are common during this phase of treatment; however, we will just take that week to week as she has subsequent counts done.

Everything else at clinic went fine. Taylor loved seeing everyone there, and she had additional doses of Vincristine and Doxorubicin. There was still excitement about 'peeing red.' Glad to see that excitement hasn't worn off yet. Following clinic, we headed to Moe's for some chicken and cheese quesadillas (one of her most frequent requests since she has been back on the steroids). Her appetite is continuing to pick up, but I am impressed at her understanding of the need to even better regulate it. She told her Daddy and me that she is trying to listen to her belly and to stop eating when she gets full. We'll see if she is able to continue with that kind of self-control as we progress through the remainder of the 21-day steroid regimen...That's a lot to ask of anyone, especially a 3-year-old, so we are also realistic. We just continue to be amazed with her understanding of the effects the medicine(s) have on her little body.

Outbursts have been manageable to date. Our most significant one today dealt with the fact that McDonald's was no longer serving bacon, egg, and cheese biscuits at 11 a.m. this morning. She wanted me to drive around and find a McDonald's that was still serving them, and I explained that it wasn't possible (in addition to the fact that we needed to get to clinic). I explained to her that everyone knows that lunchtime at McDonald's starts at 10:30 a.m. (which is a good thing when she is craving chicken McNuggets when she is on steroids); however, not such a good thing when she is craving their breakfast menu after 10:30 a.m. We got past it though, and settled on having a bacon, egg and cheese biscuit tomorrow morning. This time around, I really am trying to focus on some of the humor in the situations. It helps in staying sane.

She is sleeping right now, but I will be headed to bed shortly to be ready for when she wakes up. Thankfully, she slept through the night last night....so I am hoping that tonight is the same! Love to everyone, and we will keep you posted on her week. We are almost half way through this stint of steroids!!!

Love, Rob, Kim, Taylor, and Alex

May 28, 2007

What a weekend it has been! We are officially on Day 12 of steroids, and they have also officially kicked in...Rob and I made the decision to divide and conquer with the kids this weekend due to where we would be with steroids, and it was a good idea. Taylor and I ended up making a trip to Grandma and Grandpa's house (which was also nice so I could see the house at least once more before it was sold...what a crazy thing to see that 'For Sale' sign in the front of the house!) Taylor and I found a lot to do though to keep busy, which also seemed to distract her from eating non-stop. We went to the beach and looked for shells, played in the pool, and helped Grandma and Grandpa load the U-Haul.

Taylor's assistance with that included making sure that Grandpa loaded all of her toys and books to go to their new house.

We are back in Tallahassee, and trying to find lots of things to distract from food. It is hard to watch Taylor go through the side effects from the steroids again....the hardest being the appetite and lack of ability to sleep. She is also starting to have a little bit of an issue with some skin breakdown on her bottom, but we are keeping that in check with zinc oxide. I guess in a weird way we should be thankful. Of all of her medicines in the various phases she has had to date, the steroids have been the toughest and the ones with the most notable side effects.

On the comical side, she has had quite a craving for ketchup with all of her food this time around- the most interesting being the pancakes with ketchup on Saturday morning. Thankfully, by the time she got to the pancakes, her belly was too full to eat them; however, Mommy had the opportunity to try them. Taylor said 'Mommy, these are really good, and I want you to have one.' At the risk of setting off an outburst, it was worth it to try one bite of pancake with ketchup. While I wouldn't recommend it, it wasn't as bad as I thought it would be...

We will keep everyone posted on her progress this week. We head back to Gainesville on Thursday, and we will wrap up with steroids a week from Thursday. Hope everyone has a wonderful Memorial Day, and thank you for all of your postings.

Love, Rob, Kim, Taylor, and Alex

May 29, 2007

The past two days have been a little rough. Appetite and sleeping challenges are continuing to increase, and the steroid side effects have now also moved onto outbursts of kicking, screaming, scratching, and hitting. We've had to keep a close eye when Taylor and Alex are playing. One minute, everything can be fine, and the next...Taylor is going after her...ready to hit or scratch her. There are still good times during the day, but they are less and less (as the outbursts are more and more). The good news is that we are finishing up Day 13 of steroids today. It is so hard to watch her little body go through this, but we also know it is a very necessary part of her treatment. We are just thankful that there is an end in sight...1 week from Thursday, she'll be done with the steroids. Grandma and Grandpa are also going to be taking Alex to Sarasota tomorrow so that Rob and I can continue to concentrate on helping Taylor get through this last stretch of the steroids. It will also help to keep Alex from picking up some of the bad habits that Taylor is demonstrating to her right now....yelling, screaming, kicking, etc....

No big cravings for ketchup today....just cravings for lots of food (spaghetti, Chick-Fil-A, Moe's, oatmeal, and strawberries). We are trying to keep her busy to distract her from wanting food, but so far the only time she doesn't want to eat is when she sleeps. She has been taking more naps during the day- usually 20 - 30 minutes at a time. We think she is probably tired due to not sleeping as well at night, but again....there is a light at the end of the tunnel, so it will all be fine.

We head to clinic on Thursday, and I told Taylor that we can try to go to the butterfly farm in Gainesville if she is feeling up to it. When I asked today, she said she would still like to go, so that is good. We will keep you posted on her clinic visit this week. I just remind myself that she is a strong-willed little girl which is exactly what she will need as she continues

through this. Love to all...
Love, Rob, Kim, Taylor, and Alex

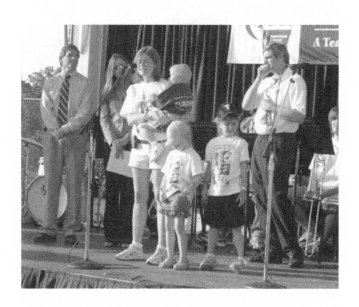

Kim Koegel

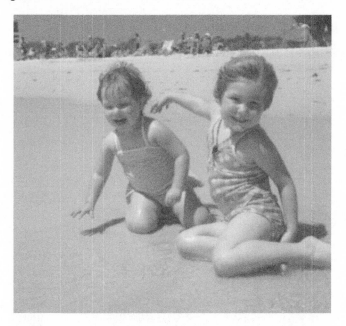

SUMMER 2007

June 1, 2007

We returned from Gainesville late this afternoon (with our suitcases still packed....which is always a good sign!) Taylor was very brave again, and did a good job getting her buddy accessed and getting all of her medicines. Today, she needed to get dosages of two of her chemotherapy drugs: Vincristine and Doxorubicin. Her counts are remaining at an acceptable level as well. Her ANC was 1008 today which the doctors were happy with. While this was significantly down from her ANC of 4000+ last week, she was still in a good range. Her doctors reminded me that she is in the midst of intense chemo, with more to come, and that we should expect to see her counts continue to drop. Her white blood cell count today was 2.4, her hemoglobin was 13, her hematocrit was 37.4, and her platelets were 130. There are still 6 weeks to go in this phase, and more drugs (and new drugs) to give, so we are just taking it day by day. Her next 2 rounds of chemotherapy treatment will require her to be in Gainesville for 4 days at a time. Those start in a little over 2 weeks. I asked her doctor today if it was an option for those treatments to be done as an outpatient procedure or if she needed to be admitted to the hospital for them. He explained that if there were any specific concerns that they would admit her; however, we could begin them as an outpatient procedure if that works better for Taylor. I explained that she seems to do better (from an environment perspective) when we are staying outside of the hospital, but that we will do whatever they think is best.

We had originally planned to head to see the butterfly rainforest today, but Taylor was not feeling up to it after clinic. She had zero energy, and told me she just needed to rest. She is also having side effects (from steroids we believe) of bad bouts of diarrhea- usually 10-12 times per day, although today it seemed to happen even more. I'm sure this is not helping with her feeling up to outside activities. Thankfully, she has been okay with wearing training pants to bed at night which helps with accidents, etc....While she found it hard to accept wearing these early on, there just really isn't a choice now. Her little body isn't able to make it through the night right now. It is very frustrating for her.

While we were at clinic today, a little girl walked in with her Mommy. I figured the little girl must have been someone's sister- as she didn't look like she was receiving any sort of treatment (i.e., she looked very healthy, had her long hair pulled back in a pony tail, etc.) Come to find out, she was 5 years old, and had been diagnosed with the same type of Leukemia as Taylor at the age of 3. She will be finishing up her treatments in August, and starting Kindergarten. I held my tears until we left clinic and were in the car (and until Taylor fell asleep), but seeing that little girl gave me so much hope. Taylor will be about the same age when she is finishing up her treatment- and will be almost through Kindergarten- but it was like fast forwarding to some sort of normalcy. When Taylor woke up, I talked to her a little bit about the little girl and "how she was brave just like Taylor, and had fought off all of the yucky cancer germs." Miss Kathryn will appreciate Taylor's response: Taylor asked me "Does she have a Germy too?" I told her that she must have a Germy (just like the one that Kathryn sent Taylor) and that her Germy must be doing a good job too!

Speaking of Miss Kathryn, she sent me this quote yesterday: "Faith is the place between the way things are and the good things that are sure to come." What appropriate timing to meet that little girl in clinic today...I think it just reinforced that statement to me, and how important it is to have faith in this journey and that God will see us through it according to his plan. I think he showed us a glimpse of the future today, and I know we will get there in time.

We will let you know how she progresses through the week...6 days and counting left on steroids. You will hear the rejoicing all the way from Tallahassee next Thursday night! Take care, and love to all.

Love, Rob, Kim, Taylor, and Alex

June 4, 2007

It is Monday evening, and it is 3 days and counting until Taylor is done with her steroids.

While the end of the steroids doesn't mark the end of her current phase (delayed intensification), it will at least mark the end of a long 21 days!

We have continued to have challenges with her huge appetite and her lack of sleep (which means lack of sleep for Mommy and Daddy too)- but we know that it will subside soon. Her most unique cuisine this week had to be the cornbread and Cool Whip from yesterday...Last night was particularly tough, as it was one of the first times (in a long time) that she gave us a hard time about taking her medicine. I ended up with a lapful of applesauce and pills, but I will admit that I probably caused it to spill! I can laugh about it today, but last night, it was pretty frustrating. Her daddy took over and was able to calm her down and get her to take her medicine. I think the problem was that it got too late and she got too tired. The past couple of days, she starts to get extremely moody by 8 p.m. So tonight- her daddy had a good plan. He gave her a bath before 5 p.m., and did medicine by 6:30 p.m....and then she had dinner, and was tired for bed. It worked well, and there were no fights about taking the medicine. I am so thankful that he and I are able to do this as a team. I know it would be impossible to get through this otherwise.

Alex is doing good, and tries to help calm her sister down when she gets upset. She will go over and pat her on the back. It is interesting to see the bond between them, and there are comical times too. In a previous entry, I meant to mention a funny story from last week's trip to clinic. Alex was with us and was playing in the toy area of the Infusion room while Taylor was getting her 'buddy' accessed. While Taylor was waiting for her chemo to get ready, she came over to play with Alex. Alex saw the tube hanging out of Taylor's shirt, pulled on it...and said 'Quack, Quack, Ducky.' Alex thought Taylor's tube was like Chemo Duck's tube, so I don't think she quite understood when I told her 'No, no Alex...we don't pull Taylor's tubes!' So I handed her chemo duck ...and she started pulling on chemo duck's tubes instead. When Taylor understood what Alex was doing, she thought it was pretty funny too.

We are taking Taylor to have her counts checked on Thursday (in Tallahassee at KidsCorner). We will keep everyone posted on the results. We know that there are still a little over 5 weeks left in this current phase, and that it will continue to be intense, but are hopeful that her counts will remain at a good level. Thank you again for all of your kind words.

Love, Rob, Kim, Taylor, and Alex

June 6, 2007

It is early Wednesday morning, and it has been a typical night in terms of restlessness, but I know the steroids will soon be over and they will start to work their way out of her system. People at work have asked me about my e-mails at odd times of the night, and I just explain that 'we don't get much sleep around here these days!' Sometimes when Taylor is awake, she is clingy, so you spend time snuggling and holding her...those times are good. Other times, she is in an impossible mood- so you just stay far away until she calms down. This gives me plenty of time to log on and stay current with work e-mails these days...

I wanted to request that everyone keep a special family in your prayers. A few weeks back, a coworker wrote me to tell me that his sister was recently diagnosed with the same type of Leukemia as Taylor. I found out yesterday that John's sister passed away Monday night. My understanding is that she had some complicating factors with infections as a result of her immune system being so suppressed from the Leukemia, and that she had been in a critical condition for the majority of her treatment. My heart goes out to John and his family, and I am just thankful that John and I were able to keep in touch over the past month about her condition. It also reminds us of how life can change so quickly. I remember reading (and sharing in a journal update I believe) an impactful quote from the book I was reading 'When God and Cancer Meet:' "Sometimes God takes the cancer out of the patient, and sometimes God takes the patient out of the cancer." While his plan may not seem clear or even fair sometimes to us, I try to remind myself that there is a reason, and that he takes us to a better place with no more pain or cancer. Please keep John's family in your prayers.

We will keep you posted on Taylor's progress this week.

Love to all. Love, Rob, Kim, Taylor, and Alex

June 7, 2007

I am not feeling like the model mom this morning, as it was a tough night with the steroids, but the good news is that today is the last day! Last night started off better than usual. Bath time, medicine, pajamas....all of that went off without a hitch. She even slept from 8 p.m. - 2 a.m. But by 2:30, she was adamant about needing to eat, so she and I headed downstairs. I made her a snack of turkey, cheese, fruit and yogurt- but explained that we were going to sit in the family room and eat, and rest on the couch afterwards. That started well,

117

and we both ended up back asleep. Then about an hour later, she woke up and was demanding more food. I know that she isn't herself and that she doesn't understand- but I know that she is constantly on the verge of making herself sick with the amount food she is eating. So I told her "No" and that she would have to wait until morning time. Well, you can imagine how that went over. She started screaming, and I was pleading with her to stop (for fear that she would wake up Alex and Grandma) and then we would all be up and miserable at 3:30 in the morning. But at the same time- I was just so over all of this, and I figured 'What is the worst she is going to do...scream? I am not going to enable this right now- she is going to make herself sick!' And I know that I am tired, and I know she is tired, and I know that the medicine is causing all of these side effects (e.g., overeating, outbursts, etc.)- but at that very moment, I had enough. I figured the entire household was probably already up from her screaming and yelling, so I just let her throw her tantrum. I went and laid back on the couch, and eventually she stopped. Somehow...Alex didn't wake up (at least that time). And then 5:00 a.m. rolled around, and we had the same scene. I told her she needed to rest a little more, and give her tummy a rest....and that we would have something to eat when the sun came up. So again- the tantrum...Mommy going to the couch to try and 'ignore' her so that she could get the tantrum out and over with- but this time Alex and Grandma woke up, and bless Grandma who came in and was able to talk Taylor off the ledge. Now that it is daytime, and I am reviewing everything in my mind, I feel extremely awful. I know that it is not her fault, and that this is not my child who is acting like this, but it is so frustrating. I just want her to be better and to be done with all of this. I am trying to remind myself that she has an amazing chance to be rid of all of these cancer germs if we can just stay the course and get through until March 22, 2009 (her end of treatment date). I have to remember that the end of treatment gets closer every day.

We are going this morning to get her counts checked at KidsCorner. Her doctors aren't requiring the count check today, but told us it was our choice as to whether we wanted to go get them done. Last night, Rob and I were chatting about whether it really matters what her counts are today (as this phase of treatment calls to keep on administering the medicine regardless of whether her counts get down to zero). I guess this phase is intended to just eradicate everything. But then I had thoughts in the back of my mind about needing to be sensitive to the fact that her counts can drop low enough to require blood and/or platelet transfusions- so we need to keep a close eye on that. I'll feel better knowing how she is tracking, so we are headed over shortly to get that done.

Well take care, and I guess I just needed to vent a little bit today. It is an emotional rollercoaster, but hopefully we will be on an upswing over the next few days as the steroids work their way out of her system.

Love, Rob, Kim, Taylor, and Alex

June 8, 2007

Thank you to everyone for your support and your kind words. I know it seems like we say that often in our journal entries, but Rob and I have constantly been amazed and are just so appreciative of the outpouring we've received. We continue to feel blessed that our jobs have also been extremely supportive as we help Taylor get through her treatment. It is a long road to get to March 22, 2009 (end of treatment date), and both the fire department and Accenture continue to understand and help us with the flexibility we need to get through this. There have been times, especially in the current phase of treatment, when one of us has had to call into work at the last minute. Today was a great example. Alex has come down with a virus of some sort, and we have to keep the kids separated to an extent. One of us isn't always able to go at it alone, and we will be forever grateful for that support. Rob also tells me that he constantly runs into folks from Leon County EMS when he is on scene at work, and that they always ask him about Taylor. It means so much, and we just really want to thank everyone for your thoughts, prayers, and concern for our family.

Taylor had her counts checked yesterday, and her ANC was 480. We expected it to continue to drop (as the doctors forewarned us), so we weren't in shock when it was down from 1008 last week. We were happy to see that her hematocrit and hemoglobin continued to be at acceptable levels (12 and 36), and her platelets were 180. With these levels, she is not in need of a transfusion as of yet, so that is good news. Her white blood cell count is at 2.4, which is not much lower than her count last week of 2.5, so we were thankful. She is off all of her medication (with the exception of her 3 day per week antibiotic) for the next week. This will allow her little body to build up its counts in preparation for some pretty intense chemo starting on June 19th. While we are anxious about the new chemo drugs that she will receive at that time, and just pray that the side effects are minimal, we know it is a necessary part of treatment...and we are starting to see a light at the end of the tunnel. She has 5 weeks left until she completes 'Delayed Intensification,' but we will get there!

So, we will just continue to say 'Thank You.' Thank you for your calls, your e-mails, the lunches and dinners that folks drop by....everything. We are forever grateful.

Love, Rob, Kim, Taylor, and Alex

June 9, 2007

What started out as an extremely trying day is now coming to a peaceful close (with 2 little ones sleeping upstairs...). Sadly, little Alex's stomach bug continued through the night and into this morning, and we took her back to the pediatrician today. Thankfully, the on-call doctor gave Alex a shot of medicine that helped the vomiting to subside. It also made her sleepy which gave her a chance to rest. While I wish the pediatrician's office would have taken that action yesterday, at least she got some relief today. In addition to being so concerned about Alex's well-being, we are also having to constantly be sensitive to Taylor's exposure to germs. Having Alex throw up multiple times yesterday and today- it didn't matter how much you scrub the floors...you are still nervous that Taylor may have been exposed to something and will therefore contract it as well. With the shot she received today, Alex was finally able to keep down some fluids and her whole demeanor improved tonight. When I first talked to the doctor's office this morning, they said they may have to admit her to the hospital if she was not able to keep down fluids throughout the day...so we are thankful that the medicine was able to help her get past that for now. Alex is such a sweet little one, and has been a trooper through everything to date- it just broke my heart today to see her feeling so down...it was good to see her feeling a little better tonight.

Taylor is continuing to 'come down' off of her steroids. It is a dramatic difference from just a few days ago- as she has little to no energy and pretty much slept the day away. Rob and I both believe that the sleep must be doing her a world of good though- and that she is catching up on about 3 weeks' worth of sleep! When she did wake up, she did have something to eat, but her appetite has gone down tremendously. We are thankful for that, as she is not continuing to overeat and then feel sick. We are hopeful that the water weight will continue to come off so that she feels back to her old self again soon. She did have some nausea and vomiting today, but we are hoping it is an isolated incident. We know her little body is going through a lot as she comes down from the steroids.

With everything going on today, it was pretty easy to start feeling sorry for ourselves pretty quickly. I took Alex on a walk this morning around the neighborhood, and had a little chat with God and told him that I wasn't sure of how many more things could add up before I wasn't able to come out of the house with a smile anymore....Then, as if it was good timing, I got home, and was chatting with my Mom who reminded me that there was a silver lining to all of this. She offered the perspective that we could have been going through this a week ago when Taylor was at the height of her steroids. With that....I took a whole new perspective on today, and was thankful that we are where we are in the process. There is always that silver lining I guess- I just needed someone to help me find it today.

Many thanks to Grandma and Grandpa for their help with the kids over the past couple of days, and for Grandma who stayed in town to continue to help with the kids and who cloroxed the house from top to bottom to try and kill whatever germs may have managed to get in here! And thanks to Angie who let me vent today when I needed to. Things are peaceful right now, so Rob and I will probably get some sleep and pray for a calmer tomorrow. Love to all, and thank you for being there for us.

Love, Rob, Kim, Taylor, and Alex

June 11, 2007

Each day gets better. Alex is feeling better again, and Taylor's demeanor continues to improve each day. It has taken longer for her to 'come down' from the steroids this time, but maybe it is also because her dosage was higher. Regardless, there is a marked difference in her behavior from just a few days ago, and it is a welcome change in our household. We have even been able to get her outside more in the past couple of days. Yesterday, we went on a pontoon boat ride with her friends Sydney, Graham, Miss Shannon and Mr. Craig. There were some bumps throughout the trip (i.e., a couple bouts of 'sea sickness'), but overall, the fresh air seemed to be great for her. Since she has never gotten sea sick before, it may have just been some left-over nausea from recent days....regardless, it has subsided, and it is yet another thing to be thankful for.

Her eyes continue to be bigger than her stomach- but now,

she just doesn't finish her meals. We are okay with that for now. It is so nice to see her appetite get back to normal and to see her begin to focus on activities other than eating.

I was talking to my Mom tonight about how quickly time can go by. As of this Thursday, we'll be half way through 'delayed intensification' (her current phase of treatment). There is still some tough chemo to go, but we are getting a little closer to 'Maintenance' with each passing day.

I've posted some new pictures tonight- some of Alex and Taylor just being silly- and one of my favorites...the girls cooking up one of Taylor's 'special breakfasts' recently. For most of the mornings that she was on steroids, she requested a 'special breakfast' which typically consisted of some sort of breakfast meat, eggs, waffles or pancakes, and something random (such as a pickle or potato chips). Ketchup was also often included in the mix.

Thank you again to everyone who has reached out to check on us and for those of you posting who remind us of how close we are to getting back to some sort of normalcy. There are so many people out there that check in on us that we've never met (in person anyway), and who continue to give us perspective on where we are in this journey. I am hopeful that we will be able to share our experience in much the same way- and to give other families the same support.

Love to all...Love, Rob, Kim, Taylor, and Alex

June 14, 2007

The past couple of days have had their ups and downs, but overall...Taylor continues to do great. She slept a good bit yesterday, but had a lot of awake time today. Strangely, she has had quite an appetite the past 2 days. Tonight she ate as if she had been starving all day long! For dinner, she had chicken, potatoes, spinach, cornbread, a hot dog, french fries, and a couple of bites of spaghetti. When it was time to go to bed she told me that I hadn't given her enough food to eat tonight. She eventually calmed down and fell asleep. She looked a little pale to me this evening, but she has continued to have good energy....we are headed to clinic on Monday evening for an early Tuesday morning start on chemo, so she will have her counts done then as well. We will just continue to keep an eye on her this weekend.

Next week will be pretty busy, but will also give us perspective on what the next 2 weeks will be like. She will be receiving her new chemo drug which will be administered on Tuesday through Friday of next week (in Gainesville). We pray that her little body continues to handle her chemo drugs with minimal side effects, and that she stays strong through this process. She and I talked about bringing her portable DVD player and her 'Barbie 12 Dancing Princesses' movie with her to Gainesville so that she can watch it at the hotel and at clinic. Thank you so much to the Sarasota County Fire Department for getting that for her. It truly makes her happy to be able to watch that movie! Sometimes when the movie is on, she dances around the family room...just like the princesses. She told us she wants to take ballet soon. I told her that we can ask Dr. Hunger about starting ballet in the Fall.

Love to all, and thanks for checking in on us. We'll keep you posted on her weekend!

Love, Rob, Kim, Taylor, and Alex

June 20, 2007

Taylor is resting peacefully tonight. It was a long day, and we both fell asleep around 10 p.m. on Tuesday night, but now I have woken up in the middle of the night and am wide awake, but a good time to update the journal too! I'm fine with just watching Taylor sleep though. There is always that part of me that worries about side effects of chemo that she hasn't received before, so there are nights when I'll lie awake and just make sure she's okay.

We arrived at clinic around 8:15 this morning to begin her

chemo regimen for the week. She received 2 new drugs at clinic today: Cytarabine (Ara-C) and Cyclophosphamide (CPM). She is also starting a 2-week regimen of a nightly pill called Thioguanine (TG). Thankfully, the doctors and nurses use the descriptions in parenthesis above, so there is no need for me to try and pronounce those drugs. As part of administering the drugs, there was a need for Taylor to stay extremely hydrated. Therefore, after accessing her buddy, they began administering IV fluids. Rob and I also had her start drinking fluids when we left Tallahassee around 6 a.m. so that we could hopefully get a jump start on the process. Her nurses had explained to us that her urine specific gravity had to be at a specific level prior to administering the dose of CPM (hence the need for so many fluids prior). I thought this was interesting as I couldn't remember the last time I had used the term specific gravity- I believe it was Physics in high school- so I needed a crash course from Rob as to what this even meant. My basic understanding is that they wanted her to reach a certain level of hydration and that is how they measure it. Following the administration of the drugs, she needed to receive another 3 hours of fluids before we left clinic. We wrapped up around 5:15 yesterday- exhausted from a long day, but a productive one. I am happy to say that she had a good day overall, and made the most of having to spend all day at clinic. We spent time watching movies, coloring pictures, talking with other little friends that were in and out- she did great. She was just so tired though. She didn't nap during the day which meant she crashed as soon as we drove out of the parking lot. That was good though because I spent the next hour trying to locate a pharmacy that carried her new medicine (TG). Nobody in the Gainesville or Ocala area carries this, but Walgreens said they could get it here tomorrow. So I called her doctor to see how critical it was if she didn't start the pills until Wednesday. I even offered to bring her into the hospital last night to get a dose there if she needed it. He said it wasn't critical, and that starting the drug on Wednesday would be fine. So, back to Walgreens where they ordered it for us- and it should be in around 2 p.m. on Wednesday.

From there, we headed to the dinner location of her choice (her favorite happens to be McDonald's when she is with Mommy). I grin and bear it as I do always want her to pick the special dinner place after her day at clinic, but we have eaten a lot of McDonald's in our trips to Gainesville over the past 5 months! We carried our picnic dinner out by the pool of the hotel though, which was nice. After dinner, she dipped her feet in the pool, but she understood that we couldn't go swimming (due to the fact that her port was accessed and can't get wet). She was fine with that though. We also spent time walking outside, and even headed across the street to the gas station for an ice cream treat. I told her I was very proud of her for walking around and getting so much exercise. She has been struggling with stairs lately, but is being persistent. She even wanted to take the stairs at clinic yesterday instead of the elevator. She just needs to hold my hand and take her time, but she gets there.

Her counts were good- up to 946! Her white blood cells are 4.4, hemoglobin was 10.2 and hematocrit was 30.9. Her platelets were also at 233, so her levels are good right now. The week off of her medicine must have been helpful in getting her counts back up for these next 2 weeks of intense therapy. We were happy to see that they were at acceptable levels. We are off to the hospital early in the morning for a lumbar puncture where she will receive additional chemo in her spine. During the procedure, they will also administer her Wednesday dose of the Ara-C, so that will save us a trip to clinic in the afternoon. We'll return to clinic on Thursday and Friday for additional chemo, and then home on Friday- a busy week, but all part of the plan. Today marks 5 months into treatment. Some days, we still can't believe it, and you wonder how you got here in the first place. But then you just keep moving! I thank God every day for the time we've had with her over the past 5 months. Love to all, and we will keep you posted on her progress here in Gainesville....

Love, Rob, Kim, Taylor, and Alex

June 21, 2007

It's Thursday morning and Taylor is helping me update the website. She helped me upload the pictures to the computer and pick which ones to put on the site. As we uploaded them, it reminded me of what a busy week she's had! There were pictures of her visit from Aunt Kathy, fishing with Daddy, visiting with Aunt Val...and then pictures from our trip to the butterfly rainforest yesterday.

Taylor had a really good day yesterday, starting with an LP early yesterday morning. I am amazed at how comfortable she is getting with the whole process- going to Pre-Op, getting fluids / 'sleepy juice' to head back for her procedure, waking up in the Recovery room....lots for a 3-year-old! She has even gotten to a point where she will ride back to the operating room by herself. For a while (and I was okay with it)- either Rob or I would ride back with her. A huge part of her feeling so comfortable are some of the amazing nurses she has interacted with over time. Every time we go to Pre-Op, she has 'Nurse Kathy' (which she also thinks is pretty neat because she has an Aunt Kathy who is a nurse too). Taylor loves seeing Nurse Kathy, and feels very comfortable with her. Once in a while, Nurse Kathy will even get smiles from Taylor that early in the morning... As part of her LP yesterday, Taylor also received a dose of Ara-C (one of her chemo drugs for this week). This saved us a trip to clinic yesterday, and gave us a chance to rest / relax, and find some stuff to do in Gainesville during our stay. Once she was feeling up to it, we left the Recovery room, headed upstairs to the 5th floor to see 'Miss Lee' (one of Taylor's nurses from when she was first admitted). Taylor likes to visit Miss Lee once in a while, and she likes to just check out the playroom while

127

we're up on the floor too. She stopped and played awhile, including coloring a picture of a butterfly that she found in the playroom. From there, we headed to Subway for lunch, and then over to the museum to see the butterflies in the rainforest. Grandma and Alex came to meet us, which was great. The girls were so excited to see each other, and hugged and hugged and hugged...The girls had fun running around the museum and playing in the exhibits...and of course the butterflies were amazing. We were at the museum for a while due to the downpouring of rain outside, but the girls didn't seem to mind. We were able to have dinner with Grandma and Alex before they headed back to Tallahassee, so it was a really good day.

Today, we are headed back to clinic for her additional dose of Ara-C, and then will stay here for another trip to clinic on Friday morning. This has been a busy week, but we are getting closer to the end of 'delayed intensification' each day! If the rain can hold off today, Taylor said she would like to go visit the 'Swamp' for a picnic....we'll see if we're able to get there. It's been pretty rainy! Love to all, and we'll keep you posted on her progress this week.

Love, Rob, Kim, Taylor, and Alex

June 21, 2007

Today was a good day, but we had a slightly longer clinic visit than we initially expected. When we got to clinic, her Ara-C was ready; however, Taylor's port was giving her problems again. We had run into some issues on Tuesday and Wednesday of this week where the nurses were not able to draw back blood from her buddy. The reason this is a concern is that there could be some sort of blockage around the line with her port, and her nurses need it to be cleared in order to effectively administer her medicine. Each day, the nurses were able to eventually clear it by either reassessing her port or by using some Heparin to loosen up whatever was blocking it. They also had Taylor change positions (put her arms up in the air, sit up straighter, lay down, etc.) Eventually, it would work. Today, it took Heparin as well as some stronger stuff (called TPA) to unblock her buddy. I told Mr. Dax and Miss Amy at clinic that we had all day, so we weren't worried about having to sit tight until we got it working again. Eventually it did, she got her Ara- C, and we wrapped up at clinic around 5 p.m. From clinic, we headed to an early dinner with the intent that this would allow sufficient time for her to eat, wait 2 hours to take medicine, and then get to bed at a decent hour. We ran into an issue however when a fire was reported on the 2nd floor of the restaurant we were eating at.....so I quickly wrapped up our stuff, paid the bill and got us walking back to the hotel. While the staff didn't seem too alarmed about it, I explained to Taylor that she should never stay in a building where someone thinks there could be a fire, and that it is always okay to leave. Taylor was bummed that we had to leave our 'special dinner' but was also kind of shook up at the prospect of a fire in a building she was in. She told me that we should call Daddy so he could help. I explained to her that the firemen in Gainesville could take care of it. We headed back to the hotel, but are in a bind now as we are 1.5 hours behind schedule for eating and then medicine, so now I will have to wake her up to take her medicine- something I am dreading, but she can't miss these doses.

Speaking of the fire department, she has been making me laugh the past few days. Being so close to Shands, we see and hear a lot of ambulances and fire trucks going by during the day. Poor Grandma made the mistake yesterday of saying 'Look at the firetruck!' Taylor was quick to correct her and tell her 'No Grandma, that is an Engine...and the other one is a Ladder truck.' It took all I had not to just laugh. She is particular about calling the firetrucks by the correct names, and each time one goes by she wants to be clear about which station it is from....'Look Mommy, it is Engine 2!' She also told me she would like to visit the firemen in Gainesville, and that she wants Daddy to take her when he comes to Shands next time. I told her that he would be happy to do that. I also told her that we should bring them cookies because it is nice to bring treats. She said we could get them some cookies from Subway.

It has been a long week, and I will be happy to head home. Having said that, it was a great moment today when we received her roadmap for 'Maintenance.' Her doctors will be walking through it with us next week, but the fact that we were handed a piece of paper that shows her regimen for the last phase of her therapy is an amazing thing to see. 'Last phase' may be misleading, as it is 22 months in length, but we are hopeful that it will be a more predictable phase and one that helps get us moving toward some more normalcy for Taylor. Time will tell, and we will continue to take one day at a time for the foreseeable future. She has amazed us to date, and is just trying to get through her next few weeks of this current phase. We'll concentrate on that for now.

Prior to signing off, I just wanted to thank everyone for their help over the past week. Thank you to Aunt Kathy for visiting with Taylor last weekend and making yummy meals for the freezer. What a help those have been! And thank you to Miss Sarah for her kind words, reminding me that we aren't walking alone through this, and her offers to help with meals. When we are home, it takes away the stress of having to figure out dinner with everything else going on....Thank you to Grandma and Grandpa for keeping Alex over the past week. She has been continuing to get the focus and love that she needs- especially when it feels like it's hard to keep that balance with Taylor needing so much attention during this part of treatment. I guess we just always want to remember to say thank you to everyone...Thank you for being there when we ask for help, and even when we haven't and you've 'just done it because you know we need something.' We are forever grateful....Love to all, and I'll post an update tomorrow night with our wrap up from this week of treatment.

Love, Rob, Kim, Taylor, and Alex

June 23, 2007

It is Saturday morning, and we are home in Tallahassee. Yesterday's visit to clinic went well, and her counts for the week ended up over 1200....Even with a higher ANC, we still need to be very careful, as her white blood cell count is down to 1.9 (from 4.4 on Tuesday). This is expected, as the chemo she had this week is doing its job of knocking all cells (good and bad) out of her body. One more week of the Ara-C and she will be done with the IV administered chemo for a bit. She continues to take a daily dose of chemo at night, and has been doing well with that. It is hard watching her have to go through all of this, but all in all, I try to remember to be thankful that she continues to make progress.

Her hair had started coming back in this last phase, but has now all fallen out again. I'm sure the chemo in this phase has caused that, but she doesn't even seem to care (or notice really). Nurse Donna told us that her hair will most likely start coming back during Maintenance, so that's good to hear. It is a blessing sometimes that she is so young! She just doesn't seem to have the cares about the side effects that us adults would!

She is off to the park with Daddy and Alex today while Mommy heads to a baby shower. It will be nice to get some time with girlfriends today....and nice for the girls to get to hang out at the park. We'll keep everyone posted on her progress next week. Love to all. Love, Rob, Kim, Taylor, and Alex

June 26, 2007

It is Tuesday evening, and Kim and Taylor are still in Hogtown. Taylor got her chemo today and all went well for the most part. Taylor's counts were extremely low and she will need a blood transfusion in the morning. The Doctors told us the new chemo would drop her counts and they did not seem concerned with low levels. Kim called and said Taylor has a lot of energy and is in good spirits. She got to play with Carson at clinic today and hang out with nurse Amy.

I apologize for the short update, Kim is much better at this than I am. Please pray for Taylor this week as her counts may continue to drop. Love to all.

Love, Rob, Kim, Taylor, and Alex

June 28, 2007

It is early Thursday morning, and we wanted to say thank you to everyone for your prayers for Taylor. Taylor received her blood transfusion yesterday morning and then subsequently received additional chemo (her Ara-C). It's been awhile since she has been transfused, but it is amazing how she "pinks up" while she gets the blood. Additionally, her blood pressure and pulse looked a lot better afterwards. Her pulse had been extremely high the day before due to her heart beating faster to compensate for the need for good blood to move through her body...There is a lot that goes through your mind when you watch your child go through things like this- but one thing I thought about yesterday was how appreciative I was that someone had donated that blood. That is on my to-do list as well...to get on a regular donation schedule at the blood bank here in town.

Taylor did great during her visit to clinic, and stayed in the play area the whole time. It's just interesting to watch kids go through this. She got 2 units of blood and her chemo while doing puzzles, coloring pictures and posing for pictures with Mr. Dax (she wanted pictures of her with all of her friends from clinic). It didn't really phase her. She was a little confused about the blood transfusion, so I explained that she needed to get some blood today as part of her medicine treatment....since that didn't sound fun, I told her we could pretend it was ketchup. She liked that better. Taylor has also been excited about coming home to Tallahassee to show Alex how her buddy looks when it is accessed. She even wanted us to take a picture...she spends lots of time looking at it in the mirror and trying to understand how it all works.

Yesterday's visit was a draining visit from an emotional perspective though. Everyone visiting clinic is fighting a battle, and everyone in that Infusion room is getting some sort of treatment with the goal of staying alive. When you think of it like that, it can make you crazy, but it's true. We have met all sorts of amazing people fighting all sorts of battles. My heart went out to a family yesterday who just received word that their son had relapsed with Leukemia ALL after being done with treatment for over 3 years. I spent most of yesterday on the drive home sobbing and thinking 'What if?'- but Rob reminded me that I can't think like that- it will not help in trying to stay positive, and he is right. I reminded myself last night that we just have to stay the course and have faith that this whole journey will turn out as it is intended to, and that we just have to take it day by day. Rob and I have consistently just try to look at short term goals- like getting from phase to phase. Taylor is 2 weeks away from Maintenance- we are going to focus on that right now.

We are headed back to clinic today and tomorrow for additional doses of Ara-C, and then they will check her counts as well. They are extremely low right now, as the doctors expected them to be. We are monitoring her temperature closely to make sure there is no sign of fever too. After we get to next Tuesday, she will have 2 weeks off of her chemotherapy which should allow her counts to rebound. That will be comforting.

We will keep you posted on her progress this week, and thank you again for keeping her in your prayers.

Love, Rob, Kim, Taylor, and Alex

June 30, 2007

Taylor and Rob got back from Gainesville on Friday afternoon. It was a good trip, but a long one as she needed another blood transfusion on Friday due to her counts continuing to fall. Unfortunately, the doctors explained to Rob that they expect her counts to continue to fall through next week, and that she may need additional blood and platelet transfusions next week. We have set up appointments here at KidsCorner for her counts to be checked on Monday and Thursday (with the likelihood that she will receive transfusions as well). While it doesn't seem like her counts could go much lower, we will just continue to be patient while the chemo does its work. I have to remember it kills the good cells and the bad cells. We are just keeping a close eye on her, and watching for fever. She is extremely susceptible right now to infection, so she is basically on house arrest for the foreseeable future (most likely the next week!) She won't mind being home for the 4th of July, as she is really looking forward to a big barbeque..(God Bless America day is what she has been calling the 4th). Grandma got her a 'God Bless America day' part set with hats and blowers, and she is pretty excited.

Thank you to Aunt Kathy who drove up to Gainesville to help with Taylor's clinic visit yesterday, and thank you to Grandma for helping with Alex so that Mommy could head into work yesterday! We are continuously grateful for everyone's help, and are always thinking about how we can turn this experience into a positive thing ultimately. I was talking to a friend yesterday about how blessed we have been by the generosity of family and friends, and that we want to be able to give back and figure out a way to help the families of newly diagnosed kids to get that kind of support. I keep on thinking about a way to set up a fund or something that would give parents an 'orientation' packet when their child is admitted- something with gift cards / certificates for hotels, gas, food, etc. There will eventually be time to focus on how all of that could come together, but I do want to figure it out someday. I just know that we were so appreciative of the outpouring of support, and want others to have that same assistance. Sadly, an illness like this can be straining on anyone's finances, and Rob and I are just blessed to have each other, good jobs, insurance, and friends and family who have helped so much. I've said before that I can't imagine what the bill (without insurance) for all of this treatment would be. I know that insurance isn't perfect, but we are extremely thankful that we have it! Well enough about all of that...

The girls and I are headed to Grandma and Grandpa's house today for a change of scenery. Their new house is really coming together, and I still have to pinch myself sometimes to remember that they really live here now. The girls love it, and have their own room at Grandma and Grandpa's- complete with their toys and own desks for coloring...it's no wonder they keep asking Grandma to have a sleep-over!

Love to all, and we will keep you posted on her progress this week. We are 2 weeks away from Maintenance, and I can't believe it's so close...

Love, Rob, Kim, Taylor, and Alex

July 3, 2007

Great news from Taylor's trip to KidsCorner yesterday. While her counts continue to be low, they are holding at a high enough level where she did not need any blood or platelet transfusions yesterday. We will continue to hope for good results from her visit this coming Thursday too, as she will be on a 2 week break from her chemo medicine starting tomorrow. This will give her body (and her counts) a chance to rebound, so we are interested to see what her counts look like on Thursday.

She and Alex are both fighting a stuffy nose right now, but we are just keeping a close eye on both of them for fever. With the exception of Miss Alex taking a tumble down the stairs this morning, everything else seems to be on the upswing in the Koegel household. Alex seems to be okay, and was just pretty shook up from the fall. She and Taylor will be spending the day with Grandma, so they are excited about that. Taylor is looking forward to 'God Bless America' day tomorrow, and is talking non-stop about a barbeque and fireworks. She already has her red, white, and blue outfit picked out.

Love to all, and Happy 4th of July.

Love, Rob, Kim, Taylor, and Alex

July 6, 2007

Taylor had a great 'God Bless America' day, complete with fireworks, a barbeque with the family, a flag cake, and visits with friends... She sang 'God Bless America' throughout the day, and even took her nap so she could stay up later for the fireworks. She really had a great time.

We had her counts checked yesterday, and they continue to stay pretty low; however, they were high enough to hold off on any transfusions right now. She will be headed to Shands on Monday for a check-up with the doctors, and we are hopeful that she continues to progress as she nears the end of this phase.

We received some sad news yesterday that a good friend passed away unexpectedly on July 4th. Mary was an amazing lady, and offered such kind words and comfort to me as Taylor has progressed through her treatment. Rob and I were over at Scott and Mary's house recently, and Mary shared with me some of her favorite bible verses that helped her get through tough times. I hope she knows just how much it meant to me that she took the time to share those with me. She will be very missed, but we all have another angel watching over us now. It is yet another reminder of how precious every moment with our loved ones is, and my heart goes out to her family in this tough time. Taylor asked me why Rob went to see Scott yesterday, and I explained that it was Miss Mary's time to go to heaven, but Mr. Scott wanted her here, so he was sad, and Daddy wanted to check with Mr. Scott to tell him it would be okay. She seemed to understand.

We will keep everyone posted on Taylor's trip to Gainesville next week. Love to all...

Love, Rob, Kim, Taylor, and Alex

July 10, 2007

We made a trip early yesterday to Gainesville, and returned with news that her counts are rebounding- slowly, but surely. The good news is that the doctors didn't feel she needed any transfusions because her counts seem to be rebounding on their own. She is still neutropenic (highly susceptible to infection) with her counts at 352 yesterday, but they are much improved over the past 2 weeks. It is amazing to us how the chemo has just knocked everything out! Her white blood cell count was up to 1.1 (up from .4 last week), and her hemoglobin, hematocrit, and platelets were all at levels where a transfusion wasn't needed. She will have her counts checked on Thursday this week, and Wednesday of next week. Assuming she 'makes counts' of 750 and 75 (i.e., ANC of 750 and platelets at 75), she will officially begin her 'Maintenance' phase on Thursday of next week. Assuming she starts next week, she will have IV administered chemo as well as a lumbar puncture on Friday, and then she will resume daily oral chemo. We are getting closer each day!

Love to all, and thank you for praying for Taylor. She continues to amaze us.

Love, Rob, Kim, Taylor, and Alex

July 11, 2007

On the eve of Taylor's 4th birthday, I realize that I am still sometimes in disbelief of where we've been over the past 6 months. Her birthday tomorrow is definitely a celebration on so many levels...but mostly a celebration of life and strength and perseverance. She is an amazing little girl. She will have her counts checked tomorrow, and we continue to hope that they rebound so that she is not so susceptible to infection.

Because she is still in the process of wrapping up her current intense phase of treatment, her birthday will be pretty low-key tomorrow- with dinner and cupcakes at home with the family- but it will be complete with 'Backyardigan' plates, napkins and goody bags. I told her that we can look to August to do something a little bigger with some friends (as her counts will be higher than they are now!) She understands, and is just excited about having cake tomorrow.

Our friend Carson, who is also wrapping up this intense phase of chemo, needed a platelet transfusion yesterday; however, he was unable to receive one here locally due to the lack of any matching platelets at the blood bank. It really made me realize just how important that donations to the blood bank are. I'd ask each of you to consider making that trip to the blood bank so that no person ever has to go without something so necessary. Carson was able to travel to Gainesville today and get the transfusions he needed, but I hope that isn't a concern for him in the future....I can't think of a better gift to give!

Thank you again for all of your prayers. Our little girl is turning 4 tomorrow- quite a milestone with everything that she has been through this year. Thankfully, she doesn't understand that it was ever a question...

Love to all, and we will post an update on the birthday girl tomorrow!

Love, Rob, Kim, Taylor, and Alex

July 14, 2007

Taylor had a very nice birthday- complete with the 'Christmas' cake that she wanted. She and Aunt Debbie made a yummy chocolate cake with white frosting and red / green sprinkles. Friends and family stopped by throughout the evening and brought her treats, and she was just so excited. She is still running around with the balloons that Miss Lori and Mr. Michael brought by.

Earlier in the day, she received some great birthday news. We went to KidsCorner to have her counts checked, and the results were an ANC of 560. This means that her counts have continued to go up, and she is getting closer to the Maintenance phase. Additionally, as her counts go up, it means that her immune system is improving. We still need to be careful, but the increase is comforting. By next Thursday, her overall ANC has to be at 750 and her platelets need to be at 75 in order to move on to 'Maintenance.'

Thank you to everyone for your prayers. All of them are helping Taylor to get better...I just know it. We will be in Gainesville next Thursday and Friday, and are just hoping for continued count improvements this week. We will keep everyone posted.

Love to all, Rob, Kim, Taylor, and Alex

July 19, 2007

Today is a great day! It is 6 months to the day that Taylor was transported from Tallahassee to Gainesville when she was first sick...but today's trip to Gainesville means the start of the Maintenance phase of her treatment. I say that with 99% confidence (although her doctors will need to confirm it today)- but when we had her bloodwork done yesterday, she 'made counts' (meaning that her ANC and her platelets were high enough to exit the current phase and start the next phase of treatment...her ANC needed to be 750 and her platelets needed to be at 75). From the results yesterday, her ANC was 760, her platelets were over 200, her white blood cell count was up to 2.2, and her hemoglobin and hematocrit were at 10 and 29. Her little body is fighting hard, and is rallying to get those counts back up!

Maintenance is a long phase, but it is the last phase of her treatment. It will last from today through March 22, 2009, and will consist of a daily dose of oral chemo (6-MP), as well as monthly doses of IV chemo, and quarterly lumbar punctures for chemo in her spine. There will be 5-day stints of steroids (but I will take that any day over those 21- and 29-day stints!) All in all, we are very excited. Maintenance means that she will return to school in late August and get to see her friends- there are just so many things to be thankful for. She is such a brave little girl!

She has had a great week too. We took a trip as a family down to 'Burn Camp' (a week-long camp that the firefighters host for children who are burn victims), and Taylor spent the day playing on the beach, doing arts and crafts and spending time with Miss Sarah Cooksey (her best new friend at the fire department!) Taylor thought the idea of getting to go to camp for a while was neat, and loved seeing the cabins and all of the fun things the kids got to do...She would have stayed all week if she had brought her suitcase! She has also spent time with friends, playing in the pool....just doing a lot of things that she hasn't been able to do in a long time. In a way, she has missed her summer...as the last 8 weeks have been extremely intense, and so rough on her little body. But that is a small price to pay for the end goal of getting rid of all of these cancer germs!

I wanted to share with everyone an excerpt out of a devotional I've been reading called 'Streams in the Desert.' Thank you so much to Lori and Michael for giving this to us- I read it as I can, and it reenergizes my faith every time I do. This particular excerpt is from the July 8th reading when it talks about a fable about the way that birds 'got their wings in the beginning.' It goes on to say that God gave birds their wings, and at first the birds considered them a burden. "For a little while the load seemed heavy and hard to bear, but presently, as they went on carrying the burdens, folding them over their hearts, the wings grew fast to their little bodies, and soon they discovered how to use them, and were lifted by them up into the air- the weights became wings....We look at our burdens and heavy loads and shrink from them, but as we lift them and bind them about our hearts, they become wings , and on them we rise and soar toward God....There is no burden which, if we lift it cheerfully and bear it with love in our hearts, will not become a blessing to us. God means our tasks to be our helpers; to refuse to bend our shoulders to receive a load, is to decline a new opportunity for growth."

This particular reading has just really stuck with me, and reminds me that Rob, Taylor, Alex and I will continue to grow from this experience- no matter how hard it seems at the moment. Love to all, and we will keep you posted on her trip to Gainesville today and tomorrow!

Love, Rob, Kim, Taylor, and Alex

July 21, 2007

Taylor and Daddy had a great trip to Gainesville. She officially started Maintenance!!! She had her dose of Vincristine (her IV chemo) on Thursday, and an LP on Friday morning (for the chemo in her spine)....and she resumed steroids and her 6-MP (oral chemo) on Friday as well. While it sounds like a lot- it is actually the same regimen she was on 2 phases ago during 'Standard Interim Maintenance.' The biggest thing to get used to again is the need for early dinners so that she has nothing to eat for 2 hours prior to taking her 6-MP. That is okay though- we are just happy to continue marching through this! Schedule will also be important as Taylor (and Alex too!) get back to school in August. She is very excited about getting back to school and seeing her friends again. She misses them a lot...

The weekend has been good so far. We had family visiting from Sarasota, and Taylor had a great time playing and visiting with them. She is also getting really good at riding her 'Hello Kitty' bike- a birthday present she received this week.

She'll have her counts checked again in 2 weeks, and we are hopeful that she will ease into this phase and continue to progress. Thank you for all of your prayers and support.

141

March 22, 2009 will get closer each day!

Love, Rob, Kim, Taylor, and Alex

July 29, 2007

It has been a good week overall...we are getting back into the swing of things with her Maintenance medicine regimen. She takes a dose of oral Methotrexate (one of her chemo meds) once per week on Fridays...so as of this weekend, she has had at least one dose of all of the medicines she is anticipated to take throughout this phase. (And we made it through this month's stint of steroids...yea!!!) We just continue to keep a close eye to make sure everything is going okay and to watch for side effects. So far, her energy level has continued to be great. We did notice a slight rash / a few red bumps by her mouth last night, but put some Neosporin on it last night before bed to help fix it...those of you who have known me for a while know that I think that Neosporin can pretty much fix anything! (So between that and salt water at the beach- not sure that the world needs much more to get better...). We'll keep an eye on it though, in case anything gets concerning.

We signed Taylor up for ballet lessons this week (to start in September). She is so excited, and would prefer to wear her leotard, tights, and ballet shoes 24/7 at the moment. Thankfully, when we bought her ballet shoes, the people at the studio told her that you can't wear ballet shoes outside. So- from the get go, that hasn't been a battle for me. She knows that when we leave the house- we have to put on our clothes and shoes!

We also took a visit to Taylor's school this week so she could see her teachers. This was her first time inside since her last day in January. Taylor ran inside and was so happy. She cannot wait to be back at school and see her friends. It was naptime, but they let her peek in on her friends through the classroom window. Taylor told me 'Mommy, I used to cry sometimes when you would take me to school, but I'm 4 now, and I want to go back to school, and I won't cry anymore.' Miss Peggy said it best when she said that 'it is amazing how everyone- even kids- appreciate things that we can sometimes take for granted.' Rob and I are both excited she is headed back to school, but are also being extremely cautious as it will be exposure for both her and Alex to a lot of things....and opens up risk for catching a cold. We'll just be careful, and we are planning on sending a note to parents to let them know to give us a call if they think their child may be sick. That will allow us to make an educated call as to whether we send the kids to school that day. Even in Maintenance, a fever will still put Taylor back in the hospital- so we will still need to play it safe and keep her home if necessary.

Her weekend has been great, and the girls have had fun visiting with Gammy and Aunt Kathy this weekend. We spent a lot of time yesterday in the pool, and they were both swimming like fish! It was great.

Taylor will have her counts checked this week, so we are hopeful that she maintains good levels. We continue to be amazed with her every day, and just think about all of the wonderful perspective we've gained along the way. Love to all, and we'll update more this week.

Love, Rob, Kim, Taylor, and Alex

August 1, 2007

Taylor had her counts checked today at KidsKorner, and we were very pleased to see she is doing great! Her overall ANC was over 2,000, and most of her counts were at levels higher than they have been in a while. Her white blood cell count was up to 3.1, her hematocrit and hemoglobin were up to 11 and 32, and her platelets were at 181. This was the first time we've had her counts checked since Maintenance started (2 weeks ago tomorrow), so I was anxious while we awaited the test results...I was happy that there was nothing but good things to celebrate!

Even with that good news, things still add up...just day to day stuff, and stresses in general- and sometimes you feel like you are hanging on by a string! We all have them though- not just Rob and I- and I constantly remind myself of that....but tonight I had a good cry...We were at Mom and Dad's for dinner...the kids were playing, and I was just watching them laughing with each other and playing so nicely- and for some reason, everything just hit me at once. Mom was right there though- my shoulder to cry on. She just held me and reminded me that everything would be okay. Sometimes, it's hard to remember that. Mom and Dad kept the kids tonight so I could get some things done, and Mom is watching them tomorrow while Rob is on shift and I'm at work. I am so appreciative of that support.

Taylor is looking forward to her weekend. Her friend Kaitlyn (and her mom: Miss Kathryn) are coming to visit from North Carolina, and Miss Kathryn is making a special 'Strawberry Shortcake" cake to celebrate Taylor's birthday. It will be great to see them!!!

Love to all, and we'll keep you posted on Taylor this week. Even with all of our stresses, I just remind myself that there is still so much to be thankful for. Love, Rob, Kim, Taylor, and Alex

August 6, 2007

Taylor had a great weekend! Miss Kathryn and Kaitlyn came to visit from North Carolina, and Miss Kathryn made the prettiest 'Strawberry Shortcake' cake I had ever seen! (see the new pictures we uploaded!). Taylor invited some friends from school and the neighborhood up to the park and had a nice little birthday celebration (a month after her birthday, but her counts are much better now than they were at birthday time!) It also gave her a chance to see her friends from school that she has missed so much. There were lots of hugs, and even some innocent little questions like 'Taylor, where did your hair go?' She looked to me to answer some of them, but she never got embarrassed or seemed to feel bad. I just explained that her medicine made her hair get really short, but that it is growing back. She told her friends that she is going to grow it down past her knees!

Taylor told me that her friend Kaitlyn told her about 'Locks of Love' where you can give your long hair to people who have really short hair like she does. She told me that she would like to grow her hair really long when it comes back, and that she can 'give her hair to someone else.' I love that little ones can have such big hearts....(and that they can have such positive influence from friends!)

In addition to Strawberry Shortcake parties...Taylor has also continued to spend time swimming and riding her 'Hello Kitty' bike. The exercise is keeping her legs strong, but she is just having a fun time doing it! It is such a stark contrast to just a couple of months ago when she had no interest or energy to spend time outside. We continue to feel blessed every day.

Her next trip to Gainesville is on the 16th of this month, and then she will be getting ready to head back to school. We will take it one step at a time, and see if she is able to handle half or full days. There is just no way to anticipate that right now.

Love to all, and we will keep you posted. Thank you for all of your continued prayers.

Love, Rob, Kim, Taylor, and Alex

August 9, 2007

Taylor continues to have a good week, and we just wanted to thank everyone again for your prayers. I had to have some surgery yesterday which is putting me out of commission for a bit- but so many folks have jumped in to help us out with the kids....thanks so much to Grandma, Grandpa, Aunt Kathy (who drove up all the way from Port St. Lucie!), Aunt Debbie....and thanks to Lori, Julie, and Angie for bringing dinner over tonight. Rob and I really appreciate it. It's been hard to just lay still in bed the past 2 days when I know there is so much I could be doing, but everyone is doing just fine. Taylor has been a very good girl, and she laid down with me today and told me she would take good care of me while I was getting better from my 'procedure.' (although she probably thinks Mommy is pretty wimpy...as Taylor has procedures all of the time!) She has been trying to keep Alex entertained as well, which is great. I just keep reminding myself that God may be throwing a lot at us right now, but he continues to bless us with the network of friends and family to help.

Taylor's energy level has remained high, and she is doing well with taking her medicine each night. Life is starting to feel more normal with each passing day. Rob took the girls up to their school the other day to participate in playtime / circle time. We figure it will be good to take them up there a few times prior to school starting. Hopefully, it will help with the transition back into school. It's hard to believe they have both been out of school for 8 months! The structure and socialization will be great for both of them, although I'm sure I will tear up just a bit when I drop them off that day...

We will continue to keep you posted on Taylor and her upcoming trip to Gainesville. Love to all...

Love, Rob, Kim, Taylor, and Alex

August 15, 2007

We are headed to Gainesville in the morning for Taylor's clinic visit. It is her first trip to Gainesville in a month (which is nice in a way!), but I am looking forward to her doctors seeing her in person and being able to assess her progress. She scared me a bit today because she started complaining of hip pain and underarm pain. This started flashbacks of January when she had swollen lymph nodes, which were a sign of the Leukemia. By tonight, she told her Grandma that her hip pain was gone- but these will all be questions we ask her doctors tomorrow...hopefully, there is nothing to worry about. I still spent extra time with her snuggling tonight at bedtime- just watching her and asking God to take good care of her. She has been such a little fighter, and all she wants is to be 'one of the kids' again...not to be different anymore.

Assuming all goes well tomorrow, Taylor and Alex will be starting school on Monday. Over the past 2 weeks, Rob and I have been taking the girls up to school for 1 - 2 hours at a time and sitting with them in their respective classes while they play and spend time with friends. Yesterday was a turning point for Taylor when she stayed inside with her 'big kid' class while I went outside to the playground with Alex. When I came back inside, she was still in 'circle time' and having a good time with friends. Rob and I really feel that the visits over the past couple of weeks will ease the girls' anxiety (and maybe ours too!) when school resumes next week. I will admit that it was hard for me to be at school and hear the coughs, sneezes or see runny noses. Even if they are harmless sneezes, every one of them resonates with you when you've been keeping your children isolated to the extent possible. I just keep reminding Taylor to use lots of Purell and to wash her hands as many times as she wants during the day.

Well, we will keep everyone posted on Taylor's trip to Gainesville tomorrow. Taylor is looking forward to the weekend, and is excited to see her Aunt Carol who is coming for a visit. We are all keeping Aunt Carol in our prayers- as she recently had surgery to address a breast cancer lump that appeared on a mammogram. She is my Grandma Sadlock's daughter...so that means she is a strong lady, and I have faith that she will be just fine...but it just reminds us all of this awful disease, and how many people it impacts.

Love to all, and we will post more tomorrow.

Love, Rob, Kim, Taylor, and Alex

August 19, 2007

Taylor's trip to Gainesville went well. We had a lot of questions for the doctors, but feel comfortable that she is fine at the moment. They checked out her lymph nodes under her arms and said that they were fine, and explained that the hip pain could possibly be a result of the Decadron (her steroids). If the pain persists, they will order an X-ray to look closer at her bones, but did not feel anything was necessary right now. That was comforting.

Her ANC was 600 which was much lower than the +2000 count just 2 weeks ago. At first I was concerned, but the doctors explained that this is expected- meaning that her counts will fluctuate during Maintenance, and that they will adjust the dosage of her daily chemo meds to keep her counts between 500 and 1500. It is so interesting to me that she can't be too high or too low! This is how the treatment works though, so we will continue to pray that her counts stay within this range. Her doctors feel she is good to start school on Monday, so we are all excited (slightly anxious too, but it's time to get this started). The girls and I stopped by their school on Friday to sign some paperwork and to see what supplies they will need for Monday. While I was there, I ran into one of the moms from Taylor's class, and she was so excited to see Taylor. She told me she had been following Taylor's progress on the website, and it just continued to amaze me how many are following her on this journey....She was also so gracious when she told me that if her son gets sick-she will not bring him to school. She said she doesn't want to risk getting Taylor sick. I wish I could have told her at that very moment how much that meant. I know that I can't protect her from every germ out there- but knowing that there are people out there who are looking out for her too....it just means so much.

I would ask everyone to keep Carson Chapman in your prayers (http://www.caringbridge.org/visit/carson-chapman). They just found kidney stones in his right kidney, and he is having to undergo treatment in Jacksonville where they have a pediatric urologist. I know that his family wants everything to get back to normal, including getting back to school...and that this feels like one more detour, but I just pray that everything will be normal soon.

Love to all, and we will keep you posted on her progress this week.

Love, Rob, Kim, Taylor, and Alex

August 21, 2007

Monday was the first day of school! It was actually 7 months to the day that Taylor was diagnosed...so in a weird way, it was appropriate to take such a big step yesterday. While it was Taylor's return to school, and her start of the Pre-K program, it was Alex's first day of 'big girl' school! All in all, it was a very exciting day in our household.

We got off to a little bit of a grumpy start, but by the time we got to school- both girls were in great moods, and did fine in their classrooms. Taylor did great in her VPK (voluntary Pre-K) class...her teachers said she listened, she played, and she took her nap. Alex had a good time singing songs, playing with toys, and painting. Alex did have a couple times during the day where she cried, but the teachers took her to visit Taylor (Tay-Tay as Alex calls her), and they were able to calm each other down...they really have a special bond.

Day 2 of school was a little tougher. Alex was fine, but Taylor cried and screamed about having to go. Let me just say thank you to all of the parents who tried to console me as they walked past my screaming child this morning. I received lots of support such as 'Don't worry, we've been there' or 'You should have seen my daughter yesterday...,' etc. Everyone was trying to make it better- and I really did appreciate that. A big thank you to the Scottsdale teachers who diffused the situation by just taking Taylor and putting her in class. They told me 'This is going to be harder on you, but she will calm down in 5 minutes.' Then they told me to call back in about 10 minutes. Of course, when I called...both children were doing just fine. I can't say enough about the teachers and staff at Scottsdale. They have been an amazing support network throughout this whole ordeal, and just continue to be there to get through these first crazy days of getting back to school!

When I got home this evening, Taylor couldn't tell me fast enough about all of the fun things she did at school today, and even asked me to take her in early tomorrow so she could spend extra time in the 'Home Living' center in class. I told her we would get there extra early...

We will have Taylor's counts checked this week, and we are hopeful that she has been able to maintain acceptable levels since last week. Love to all, and we will keep you posted!

Love, Rob, Kim, Taylor, and Alex

August 24, 2007

* UPDATE: Rob just called and let me know that Dr. Hunger (Taylor's doctor at Shands) has been talking with Taylor's pediatrician here in Tallahassee, and they are going to admit her here locally to Tallahassee Memorial. They feel comfortable they can begin to manage her neutropenic fever here, and then only transport her to Shands if the situation doesn't improve. (Neutropenic means that her counts were under 500 when they did her labs this morning). So, she will be admitted, begin receiving IV antibiotics, and then they will monitor to see if the blood cultures grow anything that indicate where the fever is coming from. We'll keep you posted.

ORIGINAL UPDATE:

Please pray for Taylor, as we are getting ready to head to Shands this morning. She woke up about 3 hours ago vomiting, and her temperature continues to rise. It is already to 102 degrees. Rob called down to Shands, and we have to have her admitted. While I know that regular admits are common during Leukemia treatment, we have not had to do this before, so of course I am scared to death. She will be admitted for a minimum of 48 hours, receive antibiotics, and they will run blood cultures to see what is causing the fever.

This came out of nowhere, as she has had an amazing week at school. She really loves it. We will keep everyone posted.

Love, Rob, Kim, Taylor, and Alex

August 25, 2007

Thank you to everyone for your guestbook entries and support- it really means so much!

Taylor slept good last night; however, she has continued to have a fever on and off....I was hopeful this morning around 3 a.m. when she woke up just pouring off sweat. I thought " Yes, the fever broke!" And it did...but only temporarily I guess. She was back up to 101.8 by 8 a.m. So, we'll continue to wait it out. Dr. Elzie (Taylor's pediatrician here in Tallahassee) came by during rounds this morning, and explained that we will need to continue to wait and see what the blood cultures grow, but that he believes if it was a bacterial infection...we would have seen something by now. So, it may be something viral....it may just be fever because her counts are low....either way, we just have to wait it out until she can go without a fever for a time period that the doctors are comfortable with. When Rob and I talk to her doctor today, we will have a better understanding of whether that is 24 hours, 48 hours, etc. Her doctors are holding off on her daily chemo medicine for now (until her counts come back up). Her white blood cell count was down to 0.4 this morning, so hopefully she will start to rebound soon.

The nurses at TMH have been wonderful, and are being extra conservative each time they come into Taylor's room. They suit up with aprons, gloves, and a mask to be extra careful about germs. They are also letting Taylor help when it is time to flush her port with the Heparin. I think they think she is too cute when she drops her little medical terms...or tells them that she eats cheese because it has protein and makes her strong.

Even with all of this going on, little Taylor is in good spirits. She is coloring a lot, and asked me to bring some of her toys back to the hospital today. She got to visit with Alex last night which was nice. Alex likes wearing the masks (and we call her Dr. Alex). She thinks that is pretty funny.

So, we will continue to keep you posted, and appreciate all of the prayers that are being said right now for Taylor. She is a strong little girl, but I will just be happy when we are past this bump in the road!

Love, Rob, Kim, Taylor, and Alex

August 27, 2007

Just a quick update, but I promise to type more later....the good news is that Taylor was discharged from the hospital last night. She had been able to keep the fever away for 24 hours....so the doctor felt comfortable with us going home. We are headed back this morning to the hospital to get counts checked; however, it was nice to sleep at home last night, and for Taylor to be able to roam freely without a mask.

Thank you to everyone for all of your prayers. We are still in need of her counts rebounding so that she can be above 500 and out of a neutropenic state, but she will be on her way- we just know it.

Love, Rob, Kim, Taylor, and Alex

August 27, 2007

Another quick update- but more to type later on when I get home tonight...

Taylor was readmitted to the hospital this morning. During her visit to KidsKorner to get her counts checked, her temp spiked to 101 degrees, and the doctors made a decision to admit her for at least the night. She is in good spirits, and there was positive news in that her white blood cell count was up to 0.7. While this number is still extremely low, it had gone as low as 0.4 this weekend. Her resulting ANC today was 60. Essentially, she has very little immunity right now- and with the fever, the doctors just want to continue to keep a close eye on her.

We will keep you posted. Ironically, it was raining this morning when Taylor and I were on our way to the hospital. She was looking up at the sky (which was dark), and said "Mommy, when will there be blue skies again?" I told her "they will be here soon...we just have to be patient." For some reason, when she asked that...I just had a feeling that we weren't out of the woods just yet, and that in a weird way- her innocent little question had a double meaning. So, it reminded me to just be patient, let God and the doctors do their work, and she will be back home with us in no time.

Love, Rob, Kim, Taylor, and Alex

August 28, 2007

Good news and bad news. The good news is that the doctors found the culprit of Taylor's fever: Salmonella. The bad news is that it is Salmonella. It took me awhile to find the correct spelling of it on the Internet, but I guess you would compare it to a bacteria that causes a bad case of food poisoning (Most of us have probably heard of it, but just never knew how to spell it- My understanding is that it is commonly due to undercooked eggs or from exposure to raw meats, etc.). The trouble is that with her counts down so low- it is tough for her little body to fight this off.

As any Mom would do, I have been beating myself up this morning about anything I cooked her the day before. Rob reminds me that it doesn't matter now and that we just need to deal with this from here. I also have to remember that she could have picked this up from anywhere- someone not washing their hands and then serving food at a restaurant where we got a 'To-Go' order....it could be anything. Regardless, everything in our house will be ridiculously well done for the mean time.

Dr. Elzie is consulting with Infection control specialists as well as other doctors to identify the best way to treat this and knock it out of her system. I guess it is a good thing that we know what needs to be treated now, but it still scares me to know that these awful germs got into her body.

She will need to stay in the hospital until this is cleared up, so we are not yet sure how long that will be. Please keep her in your prayers as her fever was up over 104 degrees this morning when I talked to her Daddy. She is not out of the woods by any means yet, but hopefully she will rebound little by little.

Love to all, and we will post more later.

Love, Rob, Kim, Taylor, and Alex

August 29, 2007

The doctors feel that the antibiotic treatment is working, and we were happy to see Taylor's white blood cell count rise to 1.9 as of this morning. This resulted in her overall ANC coming up to 453! (quite a jump from 171 yesterday). This just continues to give us faith that her little body is doing everything it can to fight this off. She is so strong. She was still having fevers as of this morning, but we are hopeful that the fever will subside. The doctor told Rob today that if Taylor can stay fever free for 24 hours, she can be discharged. Following her discharge from the hospital, she will then have a 5-day outpatient treatment of antibiotics at the local hospital.

She has had very little appetite the past few days, but we had a breakthrough last night with Miss Joan's Matza Ball Soup. Mr. Michael brought it up to Taylor's room last night, and it is the first thing of substance she ate in 3 days! When I came to stay with her this morning, she told me she wanted more soup. Thanks to Miss Lori for bringing some more back up for lunch today!!! Overall, Rob said she had a better appetite today. Thank you so much to Miss Joan!

Alex misses her sister, but I keep telling her that Tay-Tay will

154

be home soon. She has come for visits at the hospital, but we try to keep them short, as it can become a circus quickly in the hospital room...Grandma has been an amazing help with picking up Alex from school and keeping her in the evenings while Rob and I switch out at the hospital. Rob has been amazing, and has been covering hospital time while I'm at work this week. We switch off at times during the day so he can leave to get a shower or to visit with Alex....While I am up at the hospital, he and Alex get some "Daddy and Alex" time...which is nice. He is such a great Daddy.

One bit of news that we will have to break to Taylor is that we will not be able to go to Disney this weekend. We were supposed to be attending a 'Family' weekend sponsored by the American Cancer Society this weekend (where there are classes offered about Leukemia, etc.), and the kids would have the chance to go to one of the parks, have breakfast with Mickey, etc. I'm just reminding myself that Disney will be there when Taylor is better....so we will just have to delay the trip for now.

Well, we will keep everyone posted on her progress. We are hopeful for a hospital discharge soon, but will continue to be patient.

Love, Rob, Kim, Taylor, and Alex

Great news today! Taylor was discharged from the hospital! Her fever stayed away, and her white blood cell climbed to 2.6...This resulted in an overall ANC of over 1300. Needless to say, Rob and I were so thankful. It is hard sometimes when you are waiting in the hospital, and not sure what the next hours will bring...but I guess it helps you feel that much more thankful when things start looking up. She will have a Home Health nurse come to administer IV antibiotics over the next 4 days (Friday through Monday), and then the treatment will be wrapped up. While she could go back to school on Friday, we will be conservative, and keep her out through the weekend....the long weekend will give her some extra rest, and then she will be good to go back to school on Tuesday. She will resume her chemo meds tomorrow night, but at a half dose. Her doctors will then monitor her progress and let us know when to increase her dosage.

The guestbook entries kept our spirits up this week as well. Tonight, as I was reading them- I saw an update from a member of the Leukemia and Lymphoma Society's 'Team in Training.' This is a wonderful organization, and they have made Taylor an honored team member as they train this year. Sadly, we were supposed to head to an event last Friday night to talk to the team, but Taylor was in the hospital. I just hope the team knows how much we appreciate the cause that they are training for! I can't say enough about how comforting it is that the type of Leukemia that Taylor has comes with such a researched regimen of medicine, and that the doctors have a step-by-step roadmap with estimates of survival rates, etc. These things are only possible with the support raised for research, and we are so thankful for that.

Taylor is sleeping peacefully now, but is looking forward to college football starting this weekend (She is especially looking forward to the Clemson / FSU game on Monday night). She is already planning our 'tailgate' menu...although the tailgate will be in our family room this year! We didn't tell her that there was a game on tonight, or she would have wanted to stay up and watch it....she makes us laugh...

Well, I will sign off for now, but today was definitely a day of 'blue skies!' We will keep you posted on her progress...and of course whether she chooses her FSU or Clemson cheerleader outfit on Monday night. Mommy will leave it totally up to her...

Thank you again to everyone who offered to help this week. It is always so comforting to know we have a network of support around us.

Love, Rob, Kim, Taylor, and Alex

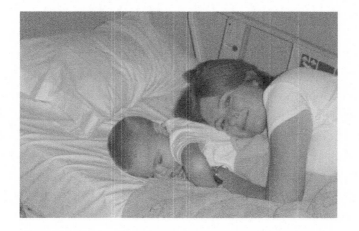

FALL 2007

It's been a busy week, but a great week overall. Taylor wrapped up her antibiotics from home health on Monday (Labor Day), and was able to get her 'buddy' deaccessed. After being accessed for 10 days, she was able to enjoy a nice bath that day (we have to be careful about getting her buddy wet when she is accessed...which makes for lots of sponge baths). Monday was also a busy day with the FSU / Clemson game. She opted for her Clemson cheerleader outfit and wore her Seminole crocs. She and Alex also made garnet and gold cupcakes as well as purple and orange cupcakes for the game. Even at her age, she has an amazing amount of diplomacy! She cheered so loud for the first half, and thought it was nice that the Tigers 'shared' the football with the Seminoles at some points during the game too. It was just nice to see her so happy...

She returned to school on Tuesday, and also started ballet on Tuesday night. She was a little nervous about ballet- especially when we walked into the lobby of the dance studio, and all eyes immediately turned to her. She may be 4, but she knows when people are staring. I can't fault people though. I know it is human nature, and I know that their hearts go out to us...but she really just wants to blend in. And I know we will get there again...slowly, but surely. Once she got over her initial nervousness about going into the ballet class by herself (with Mommy and Grandma watching through the classroom window), she had a blast! She was grinning ear to ear, and couldn't stop talking about it the rest of the night. I was surprised that we were able to get her to change out of her leotard and tights and into pajamas that night...she kept on wanting to show off all of her new ballerina moves!

We also received very exciting news today. Some of you may remember that there is a foundation called 'Dreams Come True' that talked to Taylor a few months ago about her "wish." Taylor's wish was to go see 'Dancing with the Stars.' I spoke with Amy, Taylor's 'dream coordinator' today (which by the way- what an amazing job title...making people's dreams come true!) Amy let us know that she spoke with ABC, and that we will be headed out to Los Angeles to see 'Dancing with the Stars!' Taylor is thrilled!!! You have to be 16 to be able to attend the actual 'live' show, so ABC said that she will be able to attend a rehearsal (I can understand as it would be tough to judge if small children could be fussy during a live taping). Additionally, Amy said that a rehearsal will be more laid back and give Taylor a chance to spend more time with the folks there. We can't thank the 'Dreams Come True' foundation enough. They are truly granting an amazing wish for Taylor, and she is so looking forward to it.

So- a busy week, but lots to be thankful for. Taylor will make a trip to Gainesville this coming week for her monthly dose of Vincristine, and to see her doctors. We will keep everyone posted on her progress, and thank you all again for your thoughts and prayers.

Love, Rob, Kim, Taylor, and Alex

September 14, 2007

Taylor and Rob went to Gainesville yesterday, and returned with suitcases still packed- that's a good trip!

Her counts had remained at a good level, with an overall ANC of 1100. She received her monthly dose of Vincristine, and we will start her 5-day stint of steroids when she wakes up this morning. Since her discharge from the hospital 2 weeks ago, she has been on a half dose of her daily chemo medicines, so the doctors resumed her to a full dose as of yesterday. At first, we were concerned that the full dose may make her counts drop, but (yet again), we remember we are not the ones who have studied this for years. Her doctors reminded us that they need to get as much chemo into Taylor's body as they can- and if that means her counts dropping and have to readjust again at some point, they will. It is a reality check when you remember that there are no guarantees that the cancer won't come back, and that you have to administer as much chemo into her little body as possible- even in this phase. Even though we are only 2 months into Maintenance, I think we've gotten a little comfortable (with the exception of her 1-week hospital stay) that life is getting normal again. We still need to be cognizant that her body needs to be focused on killing all of those cells...good and bad...and that normal life will resume somewhere around March 22, 2009 (her end of treatment date). Until then, we will just get comfortable with fluctuating counts and the curves that her treatment may throw us...but it is not something insurmountable.

Thank you for continuing to check in on Taylor. I will ask everyone to keep Carson Chapman in your thoughts (http://www.caringbridge.org/visit/carsonchapman). He has been in the hospital this past week, but will hopefully be returning home soon. I was writing to Carson's parents yesterday about how both Carson and Taylor continue to amaze me. When I stop for even a second to really think about everything that these 2 kids have been through in the past 8 months (and all of the other little ones out there battling this), and the gravity of it all sinks in, it scares me to death. Sometimes I think you have to force yourself to not think about it in those terms- or you would never get through the day...

Well- I better sign off. Alex will be up soon, and then the morning craziness will begin! Love to all, and we will keep you posted on her progress this week.

Love, Rob, Kim, Taylor, and Alex

September 20, 2007

It has been a full week. Following Taylor's trip to clinic last week, it was time for her 5-day stint of steroids. There were some rough patches (rougher than we've had in a few months), but we made it through, and I am happy to say that we don't have to think about those for another few weeks! We also had our first out of town trip (other than to Gainesville) in a long time....we headed up to Clemson to see a game this past weekend. Taylor and Alex had a blast. In addition to being such great cheerleaders at the game, they got to see their friends Kaitlyn and Tori at the tailgate, and got to meet two new friends: Sam and Ben. It was so nice for the kids to all run around, play, climb trees....there was lots of activity!

School went well this week, and she has had all 'green card' days so far. She also had ballet again this week...which she absolutely loves. There were a couple of teary moments this week as well....The first was when we went to the 'Build a Bear' workshop at the mall (thank you so much to Trammie for Taylor's gift card to make a bear!). Taylor decided to make a stuffed hippo there, and she got to pick out a heart to go inside. She picked a purple heart and handed it to the lady. The lady said "Oh, you picked one of our purple ones. For every purple heart, we donate $1 to childhood cancer research." Well, you can imagine how that struck me. It was just so appropriate that she picked that one...And then of course, there was a conversation last night that Taylor had with her Daddy. While they were coloring together, she told him that some of the kids at school were being mean to her and telling her she looked like a boy because of her short hair. She said it really hurt her feelings. Now, of course, as her parents, it breaks your heart to hear that...and we also understand that 4-year-old kids don't really mean anything hateful by it....but your heart still breaks. So, Rob talked to her about it, and told

161

her she didn't need to be sad. I'm sure he told her lots of wonderful things including that she is beautiful and that her hair will be long again soon...So then today, I headed off to the mall at lunch time to pick out pretty pink, purple, and sparkly hair wraps for her...she was very excited. I know that it will all be a memory soon, and her hair will be long. While I'm sure some of these things are tough on Taylor....there is not a lot we can change about it, so we tell ourselves it will help her to build character in the long run...

I do want to say a special thank you to the Sarasota County Fire Department who is hosting a 'Family Fun Day' this weekend in Taylor's honor. We are headed down tomorrow night to be there for the Saturday event....and we are just so appreciative of their continuous support. We are so looking forward to seeing everybody down there!

Well, I am going to sign off for the evening, but I did want to mention something I had read about. I'll verify it and post again this weekend, but I believe that on Monday, 9/24, in honor of childhood cancer month (September), Chilis is donating their proceeds from that day to St. Jude's. So, consider going to Chilis if you dine out on Monday....it is going to an amazing cause!

Take care, and we'll keep you posted on her progress.

Love, Rob, Kim, Taylor, and Alex

September 29, 2007

It is late Friday night / early Saturday morning, and we are thankful for another good week. In addition to a busy week of school, ballet, and a trip to Sarasota, Taylor also had her counts checked (and they were at 1400 overall!). So, we continue to count our blessings, including the network of family and friends that are continually there to support us.

Our trip to Sarasota last weekend was just amazing. I can't say enough about the Sarasota County Fire Department, and how honored we were that this year's Family Fun Day was to benefit Taylor. It was great to see so many people out at the park having a good time that day....Thanks again to Jason and to everyone who helped make that day happen.

And of course- one of the most exciting events of the week was the season opener of 'Dancing with the Stars!' Taylor was so excited it was back on, and is very excited about her upcoming trip! We recorded all 3 nights of the show this week...so she can watch it over and over again...and pick her new favorite contestants. Right now, she seems to be a fan of Sabrina and Jane. I am still in amazement of her dream coming true, and the fact that we're going out to California....thank you, thank you, thank you to 'Dreams Come True.'

We'll keep you posted on her week. She continues to amaze us. Love to all.

Love, Rob, Kim, Taylor, and Alex

October 10, 2007

What a week! Taylor had a great week, including a wonderful family trip to Daufuskie Island in South Carolina for the Lyles-Sadlock wedding....It was an amazing time. We had her counts checked the night before we left, and everything looked good. Her overall ANC was over 2,000, and she had good energy....so she was ready to go!

We left early Friday morning, and headed to Savannah where we took a ferry over to Daufuskie. The island was ideal for a wedding / family reunion.....with lots to do, including playing in the pool, beach time, finding shells, visiting the horses at the equestrian center....and then of course all of the wedding events! Taylor loved everything about the wedding, and danced the night away. I think she was practicing all of her moves for her upcoming 'Dancing with the Stars' trip! She especially loved the bride (Miss Julie), and gave her hugs every chance she got....The wedding weekend was great, and the bride and groom looked so happy. Taylor told me yesterday that she would like to go visit Miss Julie and Mr. Brian very soon. I told her that we need them to at least get back from their honeymoon first. She was okay with that!

Thanks so much to Aunt Peggy and Uncle Joel who came down to Daufuskie this weekend to visit, and to help sit with the girls when the wedding festivities were later in the evening (this also gave Mommy and Daddy a chance to hang out and visit with family!).

This week continues to be busy, with a trip to Gainesville on Thursday and Friday for IV chemo (Vincristine) and spinal chemo (her lumbar puncture). She will also resume steroids this weekend, and will be getting ready for her big California trip....she is excited about getting to see Miss Jane and Miss Sabrina! She also likes watching Miss Marie dance. We recorded the 'Results' show from last night, and haven't seen who went home yet....so I'm hoping those 3 are still there!

We continue to feel blessed as Taylor progresses through this treatment. We still just take each day at a time, but I think this weekend was even more treasured because of our new perspective on everything. As long as she was up for it (and behaving!), we wanted her to experience all of the fun of the wedding, and dancing all night under the stars....and she did. We didn't rush through the weekend, we didn't watch the clock when we were looking for shells on the beach or taking time to pet all of the horsies at the barn....we just let the girls enjoy themselves, and just soaked it all in. Lots of good memories....

Love to all, and we will keep you posted on her trip this week.

Love, Rob, Kim, Taylor, and Alex

October 11, 2007

Rob called earlier with good news from clinic....Taylor's counts were at 1260, including counts of 11 and 31 for her hemoglobin and hematocrit. This makes us feel comfortable as she gets ready for her upcoming 'Dancing with the Stars' trip. She also had her IV chemo today (Vincristine), and will have her lumbar puncture first thing in the morning.

She is having a good trip with Daddy, including a date to watch the FSU / Wake Forest game tonight. As I type this, FSU may need some extra cheering to get through the 4th quarter....I'm sure Taylor is asleep already though....so maybe the Seminoles will hear her cheering in her sleep.

Alex, Grandma, and I headed downtown tonight for the 'Light the Night' walk for the Leukemia and Lymphoma society. Our friend Carson had a team there tonight, and it was great to go see him and his family. Seeing everyone there also reminds me of just how many people this awful disease impacts. Sometimes, it is very emotional to walk into events such as the one tonight. It reminds you of everything going on, and you get sad, mad, and appreciative all at the same time. That may sound confusing, but it is something I've noticed over the past 9 months. You get sad because you wonder 'How did we get here?' You get mad because you wonder 'Why is Taylor having to endure this?' and then you are appreciative because you see the outpouring of support from everyone participating, and know that every dollar raised is helping to fund the research that is helping your child get better. And then I always remember that God has a bigger picture in mind that I can only hope to understand someday.

I had the opportunity to meet some of the 'Team in Training' members tonight as well. These are folks who are raising money to run in a marathon for the Leukemia and Lymphoma society. I got a little choked up when talking to one of the women, but I managed to get out "Thank you for running for my daughter." If I hadn't felt like I was going to burst into tears at that very moment, I would have gone into much more detail about how much I appreciate that she continues to train and motivate others to train so that money can be raised for this valuable research.

We will keep you posted on Taylor's progress this week, including how things go during the upcoming days as she resumes her steroid regimen. These various medications are just part of life now. Sometimes I still can't believe that we are almost 9 months into this journey.

Love to all....

Love, Rob, Kim, Taylor, and Alex

October 14, 2007

Day 1 of Taylor's dream trip was great! We were up bright and early at 4:30 to get the day started. We had a little scare when Taylor woke up not feeling well. She threw up, but had no fever, and perked up pretty quickly. We were ready to stay home if we needed to, but with no fever, and everything seeming okay...she had some Zophran, and was ready to go. Thanks so much to Mr. Craig for getting us to the airport on time....and for Grandma who came to stay with Alex that early! (and thanks to everyone just taking care of stuff while we're gone...housesitting, etc.)

The plane ride went well, and we arrived in LA at 11:30 (California time). We got our luggage, picked up the rental car, and then it was time to explore the big city and get to the hotel! Our hotel is right off of Hollywood Boulevard, so there is a ton to do. We spent plenty of time walking up and down Hollywood Boulevard, and taking in the sights...including all of the folks dressed up as various characters. Rob and I had been here once before, but it was adorable to see Taylor take it all in. I think she was trying to process how Batman, Spiderman, Barney, SpongeBob, Tigger, and Darth Vadar all managed to end up at the same place. She posed for some pictures with them, but then we had a serious discussion about 'Stranger Danger....' and that she shouldn't be so willing to run up to Batman on Hollywood Boulevard....it will make for a fun memory to tell her about.

Well, today is her big 'Dancing with the Stars' day....so we will be off to the studio around lunchtime. We will have an opportunity for some pictures, so I will post them as soon as I can! She is so excited, and has been looking for Jane, Sabrina, and Julianne since we got off the plane.

Love to all, and thank you again to 'Dreams Come True.' I can't even imagine how memorable today is going to be. Love, Rob, Kim, Taylor, and Alex

October 15, 2007

Yesterday was the day of a lifetime....Dancing with the Stars was just amazing! Thank you so much to Miss Sandy (our contact who was with us through the entire rehearsal). Taylor absolutely adored her, and she made sure that Taylor had a 'dream' experience!

Our trip to the studio started a little after 2 p.m. (when Taylor woke up from her nap). We arrived at CBS Studios, met Miss Sandy, and headed into the 'Dancing with the Stars' studio. When we walked in, the first thing we saw was the chandelier (that you see on TV), and then we turned the corner and saw the whole set! It was so awesome! Jennie Garth was practicing at the time, and the camera crew was practicing the various shots and angles for tonight's coverage. We stayed to watch nearly all of the celebrities- only missing Miss Marie and Mr. Floyd (at 10 p.m. Eastern time...Taylor was nearly falling asleep!) All of the celebrities were great, but the absolute best were Julianne and Helio. Helio happened to be sitting behind us (which I didn't notice at first), and just started up a conversation and asked me 'How old is she?' And when I turned around and saw who was asking, I thought that was pretty neat! He started talking to Taylor and playing with her, and said 'We should get a picture when Miss Julianne gets here.' And then Julianne showed up, and was giving Taylor big hugs. The most precious moment was when Taylor said 'Mommy, can I give them 2 of my bracelets?' So I gave Taylor 2 bracelets, and she gave them to Helio and

Julianne who wore them the rest of practice. And it didn't stop there- before they left, they came by again and talked with her for a while...Taylor told them she gave them a '12' for their dance (Since there weren't any judges there yesterday, Taylor took on that role). She said they were better than a '10.' I agree....Tony (Miss Jane's partner) was also amazing. He took Taylor out on the dance floor and was playing peek-a-boo which just had her laughing hysterically.

Another one of Taylor's favorites was the snack table. There was a huge table with every candy imaginable...and granola bars, chips, drinks, etc. That may have been one of the things she remembers most! Miss Sandy brought her a T-shirt, a signed picture from the whole cast, and then the costume department also brought her a special jeweled bracelet.

It was something that we'll all treasure forever...and Rob and I know that Taylor is just too young to totally understand how unique today was, but we know she had a great time. She told us the other day when we arrived in Hollywood- "This is my dream, and we are really here."

I can't say enough thank yous to Dancing with the Stars and Dreams Come True. Yesterday is something we will never forget!

So, everyone make sure to watch Dancing with the Stars tonight and cheer them on....all of them were just amazing. We'll post more later, as we are off to Disneyland for the day.

Love, Rob, Kim, Taylor, and Alex

October 19, 2007

We arrived back in Tallahassee late Wednesday night. What a trip! After our exciting date with Dancing with the Stars, we made a trip to Disneyland on Monday, and then did some additional sightseeing in LA on Tuesday (Santa Monica Pier, American Girl Cafe, Beverly Hills, etc.) I think we packed in as much as we possibly could while we were there!

Disneyland was really fun, and we were so proud of Taylor

for going on the Matterhorn (I guess you could call it a bob-sled rollercoaster ride). She surprised us when she said she wanted to go on it (because it looked pretty intimidating for a 4-year-old), but we've learned that she has become more fearless over the past 9 months in general! We spent the entire day there, and wrapped up just before closing time at 8 p.m. As tired as we were, we still made sure to tune in to Dancing with the Stars when we got back to the hotel. It was so crazy to see all of the dances that we saw rehearsed. We had seen each one so many times that we knew what was coming next! That was really neat.

Tuesday's sightseeing was great too. After a short detour to Walgreens (we were short on 1 day's supply of Taylor's steroids), we headed to Beverly Hills to drive around and to mail some postcards to family....we wanted to make sure to send them from the 90210 zip code...

Then we headed out to Santa Monica pier. When Taylor heard that California had a beach, she wanted to see it. She had a good time at the pier, and even rode the ferris wheel (that took some more convincing than the Matterhorn, but once she got up in the sky, she really liked it). She wasn't quite sure what to make of the beach, as the beach that is right by the pier has a lot of garbage that washes up. She thought that was pretty yucky, and said that Florida beaches are prettier. We explained that California had some nice beaches too....and that if we saw another one, we'd stop there too.

From Santa Monica, we headed to the American Girl Cafe in "The Grove." For those of you who have heard of 'American Girl dolls,' you know how a little girl's eyes light up walking into one of these stores. The neat thing about the LA store is that they have an actual cafe where you can have lunch or tea (with your doll included at the table in her own high chair of course). We ate outside on the balcony, and it was just the perfect setting. Rob opted for a sandwich and walking around the other shops, and said that we should do a "Mommy / daughter" lunch. It may have been all of the pink that scared him off....but he came back as Taylor and I were on our dessert course (which included chocolate mousse desserts in little flower pots, heart shaped cakes and star shaped cookies). We had a great time, and I would highly recommend it if you are traveling with a little one out in LA.

After our trip to The Grove, it was Taylor's nap time, so while she slept- Rob and I took the opportunity to do the sightseeing that Taylor could care less about (e.g., driving around Beverly Hills looking at pretty houses, finding Gene Simmons' house, searching out where OJ's house used to be....) I know- we were acting like tourists, but you can't be out there and not do these things!

We flew home Wednesday....the only incident being Mommy's mistake of suggesting we wear our matching blue T-shirts... The problem was that she got a few comments such as "What a cute little boy." This crushed her...and I immediately pulled out a pink shirt we were carrying as extra. I should know better, and felt just awful- because she is still bringing it up: "Mommy, why did those people think I was a boy?" From now on- it is as much pink as possible.

All in all, our trip was just amazing. I will admit that I was nervous at first when I realized the timing of the trip coincided with Taylor's monthly steroid stint. I will say that having a child on steroids in California can be a little expensive (when she wants to order everything on the menu, and then decides that she's not really hungry at all!)....but we got through it. There were a couple of meltdowns that were frustrating, but we got through those too. To the extent that we could, we just tried to give her a trip with enough memories for a lifetime. We are just hopeful that she will have lots of years to make even more memories. As each day passes, I know that we get closer to the end of treatment, but I am still coming to terms with knowing that the worrying will never stop.

Thank you for all of your posts, and thank you for checking in on Taylor's dream trip. As with any child going through this, you just want to give them the world, and hope that it takes some of the scariness and tough times away that go along with their treatment.

Love to all, and we will keep you posted.

Love, Rob, Kim, Taylor, and Alex

October 25, 2007

Just a quick update...Taylor had her counts checked yesterday, and they came back low. Her overall ANC was at 160, so she will be taking it easy for a bit.

When we talked to her doctors last night, the direction was to hold on her daily chemo for now, and then they will tell us when to have her counts checked again. Rob or I will most likely talk to Shands again today to understand when she should have her counts checked again to see if they have rebounded. We also have to be extremely careful about fever right now, as any fever will require a 48 hour admit at the hospital.

We will most likely hold her out of school for a couple of days too- just to exercise some cautious judgement...and to keep her extra isolated.

She's a tough kid though, and I'm sure she will rebound in no time. My heart just breaks for her, because she is acting fine, and is in good spirits....but we will have her on house arrest for a few days. I guess this is just how you have to roll with the punches through the course of treatment.

We will keep everyone posted, and thank you for your thoughts and prayers. She is already 9 months into treatment....

Love, Rob, Kim, Taylor, and Alex

October 30, 2007

Taylor's counts are up! She had her counts checked today, and her ANC was up to 820. Her white blood cells were up to 2.1, her platelets were up over 190, and hemoglobin and hematocrit were up too. This was a relief, as she has also been battling an ear infection since last Thursday. First, her counts came back low on Wednesday, and then after she started complaining of ear pain, I took her into her local pediatrician on Thursday. Many thanks to Dr. Martin who coordinated closely with Shands to identify the most appropriate antibiotic / course of treatment, and also helped potentially prevent a fever that could have put Taylor in the hospital. So, between this antibiotic from last week, her weekly course of Septra (another antibiotic), and a few days of house arrest, she was more than feeling up to returning to school yesterday.

I'm sure that Taylor's friend 'Germy' is also a key part of her counts rebounding. He has sat faithfully on her bureau to keep watch over her and to eat all of the bad germs that have come her way. (Thank you Miss Kathryn:)

The girls are looking forward to Halloween, and we have spent some fun times over the past couple of weeks visiting the pumpkin patches around town, and getting the house decorated. Rob and the girls have the house looking pretty scary in preparation for tomorrow night....and Taylor stayed up a little late tonight to help with the finishing touches on carving the pumpkin. The girls also helped me make some scary witch cupcakes and lollipop ghosts....so we've had a good time getting ready for tomorrow! I definitely think there have been moments (as there were at Easter) where I try to make sure that we are doing EVERY thing we can to make the most of a given holiday. I continue to tell myself that Taylor is going to be just fine, but you still find yourself making time (that you may or may not have always made in the past) to make sure you soak in the activities of the holidays. I just want her to have such special memories and to make as many memories as possible. It's probably not a bad idea to live life like that regardless- it shouldn't take a life-threatening illness for all of us to remember the simple pleasures of doing things like visiting the pumpkin patch and picking out your Halloween pumpkin....

We will post some pictures of the girls in their costumes (they are both going as the 'Tooth Fairy'...Taylor's idea), and we will keep you posted on her progress this week. She and I will travel down to Gainesville next week for her monthly clinic visit, which means her steroid stint is fast approaching (wow, that got here quick again!) On that note, I have been praying the past couple of days for God to grant me more patience. I have found myself losing my patience very quickly over the past week, and raising my voice more than I usually do, and it makes for such a stressful environment! So, I am trying to take a deep breath and tell myself to put things in perspective, and dig deep to find that patience! Before I wrap up this long post, I wanted to share another excerpt from the 'Streams in the Desert' devotional that I still try to read as I have time! (Apologies, but this is such an amazing book, I have to share these from time to time...) This is from the October 27th reading: "Stand up in the place where the dear Lord has put you, and there do your best. God gives us trial tests. He puts life before us as an antagonist face-to-face. Out of the buffeting of a serious conflict, we are expected to grow strong. The tree that grows where tempests toss its boughs and bend its trunk often almost to breaking, is often more firmly rooted than the tree which grows in the sequestered valley where no storm ever brings stress or strain. The same is true of life. The grandest character is grown in hardship."

I can't tell you how many times that reading the daily messages in the devotional have helped me feel comforted. It is amazing how your faith can continue to grow, even when times are tough...

Take care, and we will keep everyone posted.

Love, Rob, Kim, Taylor, and Alex

November 1, 2007

Just a quick update, but wanted to post some pictures from Halloween. The girls had a blast, and I was so happy that Taylor was healthy (i.e., counts are up and not in the hospital), and could enjoy Halloween with her friends. Taylor and Alex had some fun at their school parade / party yesterday, and then it was time to go home and visit friends...and get the trick or treating started!

We'll keep you posted on her progress this week. Thank you again for all of your postings, love, and support.

Love, Rob, Kim, Taylor, and Alex

November 5, 2007

Just wanted to post an update to let everyone know that Taylor continues to have a good week...she will head down to Gainesville this week with her Daddy for a checkup and to see how her counts are doing since she resumed her daily chemo. She has lots of energy (As I type this, she is currently bouncing around the room dancing and singing to Hannah Montana). She and Alex love to dance to the 'Best of Both Worlds' song...(Those of you with young kids know what I'm talking about!)

Taylor also had her first interview today. A local TV station wanted to cover a story about her trip to 'Dancing with the Stars.' We were very flattered that they wanted to talk to her about it, but weren't sure how Taylor would react. I warned the reporter that she might be kind of shy, so I asked her if we could meet somewhere that Taylor felt more comfortable...so we had her meet us at the park. Taylor ended up not feeling like talking much, but that was okay. The reporter had a chance to talk to Rob and I, and got some footage of the kids playing. It will air next week, so we'll see how that goes.

Things seem to be going well for the moment, so we will continue to be happy about that. We'll let you know how things go at clinic this week...Thank you again for all of your love, support, and postings. They continue to mean so much!

Love, Rob, Kim, Taylor, and Alex

November 8, 2007

Taylor had a good trip to Gainesville today. Her ANC was over 1,000 and the doctors are resuming her daily and weekly chemo doses to 75%. When Rob was relaying this to me, I was already trying to assess how the pill cutter was going to have to factor into slicing and dicing the pills to add up to 75%, but then he quickly explained that it will mean giving her a full dose for 4 days and a half dose for 3 days... whew...that was a relief- no difficult slicing and dicing :)

Taylor also received Vincristine today (her IV chemo) and the doctors rechecked her ears to make sure the infection from a couple weeks ago continued to stay away. She also had a flu shot. This was very interesting to me, but I feel so much better knowing that she is covered for whatever strain(s) the flu shot is intended to cover. The risk of her catching the flu is obviously a bigger scare than the risk of any side effects of the flu shot....so I was glad that they were able to give that to her today.

Other than that, we just keep taking everything day by day. While Rob and I just wish we knew that everything will ultimately be okay, we just have to take it one step at a time. Before we know it, Taylor will be 1 year into treatment, and then we will just continue to take baby steps as we get through the remaining months...She asked me the other day if there would ever be a day where she wouldn't have to take cancer medicine anymore...I told her that by her 6th birthday- she would be all done. She then said "You mean I'll be able to have dinner and then have a snack even after that? " (Meaning that she won't have to worry about not eating after dinner in order to accommodate for her medicine doses each night). I told her "Yes sweetie. You'll be able to have snacks in the evening." She was thrilled. In her mind, this is part of what she is processing!

Love to all, and we will keep you posted on her progress. Love, Rob, Kim, Taylor, and Alex

November 13, 2007

Taylor's story about her trip to 'Dancing with the Stars' aired on our local TV station tonight. I received a call from ABC about an hour before it aired, so we were very excited...and rushed into Grandma and Grandpa's house to make sure we could set the DVR to record! It is currently posted to their website too. The link to the story and video is as follows:

http://www.wtxl.tv/global/story.asp?s=7349577

I'm not sure how long the video stays posted to the site, but if you are searching for the article, the title of it is 'A Local Girl Gets To Dance With the Stars.'

Taylor didn't quite know what to make of seeing herself on TV, and after watching it a couple of times, she was okay with it. I think that it was a little overwhelming for her at first (and confusing) to see all of us on TV. Alex thought it was pretty neat though- she kept on saying "There's Tay-Tay. There's Tay-Tay."

It has been a good week otherwise. We had a slight scare on Friday morning (following her trip to Gainesville) when Taylor's temperature began to rise. It got as high as 99.7 degrees (too close for me to the 100.5 degree threshold that pushes her to a hospital stay). So, I picked her up from school just to keep an eye on her, and her temperature eventually came down, and held steady at 97.9 degrees for the remainder of Friday. Our assumption is that it could have been a reaction to the flu shot from Thursday, but again- it could just be some sort of random fluctuation too. We just continue to roll with things like this, as I'm sure we will have to for the foreseeable future.

We had a good trip to Clemson for the football game too- although the trip definitely had its moments. Taylor had a couple of meltdowns that were extremely frustrating, but sometimes you don't know if it's the steroids or being 4....so again, you just try to do the best you can. I will admit though, it becomes very tiring! The trip overall was great though, and we were able to spend some very nice time with friends. Taylor was able to see her friends Kaitlyn and Tori, and then she had the chance to stay at her friend Charlie's house in Atlanta (with Aunt Kim and Uncle Mike).

Taylor is looking forward to the holidays, and I'm sure the holidays will mean that much more to us this year. As I write this, it reminds me that I will need to schedule her appointment to have her counts checked sometime next week before Thanksgiving too!

We will keep you posted on her progress. Thank you again for your love and support. She is such a strong little girl...

Love, Rob, Kim, Taylor, and Alex

November 21, 2007

Happy Thanksgiving to everyone! It is definitely a time for us to reflect on all the things we can be thankful for...even in the midst of the tough times. We were extremely thankful to have Taylor's counts come back so good today. She had her labs drawn yesterday afternoon, and the hospital called me with results today. Her ANC was 1270, with a white blood cell count of 3.1 and platelets over 231. Her hematocrit and hemoglobin were also at a comfortable level (11.3 and 33.2). So I was very happy to get that call today from the hospital. Now we are just awaiting some feedback from her doctors at Shands as to how we should adjust her daily chemo. She is currently at 75% of her daily dose (due to tweaks they are trying to make with her dosage and her counts being so low a couple of weeks back). Not sure if they will resume it to 100% or just up it slightly, but whatever the answer, we are just happy to be home for the holiday.

With the exception of trying to heal from a split lip from

last Friday, Taylor has had a good week overall. She has had good energy and a very good appetite. She also did her first radio interview yesterday with 107.1- a local radio station that wanted to hear more about her trip to Dancing with the Stars. Mr. Troy and Miss Blythe (the morning co-hosts) were just wonderful, and Taylor warmed right up to them. It was so nice of them to want to hear more about Taylor's story, and we are so appreciative of the work that they regularly do to raise awareness for the Children's Miracle Network (which raises money for Shands).

We hope everyone has a wonderful holiday tomorrow, and cherishes the time with family and friends. We are thankful for all of you and the fact that you continue to check in on Taylor and her journey through this awful illness. We are thankful for your love and support and will keep you posted on her progress this week.

Love, Rob, Kim, Taylor, and Alex

November 28, 2007

It will be an exciting morning when Taylor wakes up....Today is Alex's 2nd birthday, and Helio and Julianne won 'Dancing with the Stars!' She was already on Cloud 9 about Alex's birthday, but Miss Julianne and Mr. Helio winning will put it over the top.

Actually, Rob and I were happy to see them win last night as well. They were so kind to Taylor when we were in California, and we really appreciated the time that both Helio and Julianne spent with her, talking, playing, posing for pictures, etc.

Taylor was my big helper last night...helping me get Alex's gifts wrapped and she made her a pretty card too.

It has been a good week. We are still trying to coordinate with Shands about any changes to her medicine dosage, so hopefully I am able to make contact with them today. We will be in Gainesville next week for an appointment, but still want to coordinate now so that Taylor is getting every bit of medicine she needs.

She had a great Thanksgiving weekend, and she had a great time decorating the house for Christmas. She and I decorated the tree, and it was so much fun. She wanted to know the story behind every ornament on the tree, and had 'the perfect place' for every ornament (sometimes 2 and 3 on a branch....), but it looks great. Every day she asks me "Is Santa coming tonight?" I keep on explaining that there is still a while to go, but that he will be here before we know it...

Love to everyone, and we will keep you posted on her trip to Gainesville. She'll get her IV chemo (Vincristine) next week as well as resume her steroids for 5 days....It feels like that steroid stint comes up pretty quick, but then I remind myself that with each stint of steroids- we are one month closer to March, 2009 and her end of treatment date.

Take care.

Love, Rob, Kim, Taylor, and Alex

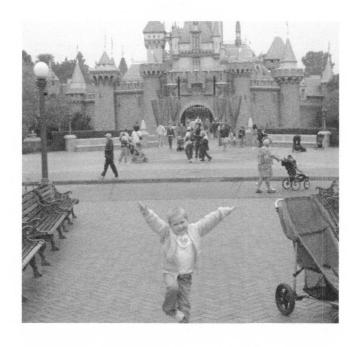

Kim Koegel

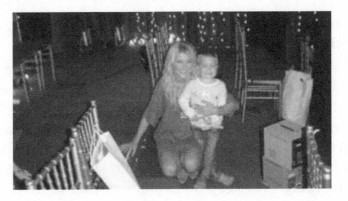

WINTER 2007

December 8, 2007

It has been a busy week, complete with her monthly trip to Gainesville. Her checkup went well, with an overall ANC of 1944. The doctors were happy with her progress, and have increased some of her chemo dosage to get closer to the 100% dose she was at previously. She had her IV chemo (her Vincristine) and resumed her steroids for 5 days....(we are on day 2 today!) When we go back next month, she will have a 2 day visit as she will also need to get her spinal chemo (her lumbar puncture) as part of that visit. As I was sitting with her at clinic, I could hardly believe that we are going on 1 year of treatment. Chemotherapy seems so routine now, which is interesting- you just come to accept it as part of the new normal we've come to know. Overall, she continues to handle the chemo well, and just had one bout of an upset tummy on the drive to Tallahassee. She had a restless sleep Thursday night, but when she woke up on Friday- she was bouncing off the walls. We feel very blessed.

Taylor had a full week, including helping to host Alex's 2nd birthday party (a Mickey Mouse party) and riding in the boat in the Christmas parade last weekend. She always loves being a part of the Springtime and Christmas parades, and especially loves getting to play with all of the kids who ride on the boat during the parade. It was a great time!

She and Alex also went to a Christmas party last night with her Daddy and I. She had a blast playing with the other kids there, and I was very proud of her for not fussing about not being able to eat any snacks there. I think playing with the other kids kept her distracted, which was nice....I know it must be hard for her to have to turn down cookies and other treats in the evening at a Christmas party, but she can't have anything on her tummy for 2 hours prior to taking her medicine. She knows that someday that will be different, but for now it just is what it is.....I am proud that a 4 year old handles that part as well as she does.

We will keep you posted on her progress this month. She is so looking forward to Christmas and has asked Santa for a pony and a house. God bless Santa who helped to clarify those requests for her...he said 'Oh, so you want a doll house and My Little Ponies?'...and she said 'Yes.' So, that alleviates the concern of having to board a pony anytime soon!

Love to all, and we will post more this week.

Love, Rob, Kim, Taylor, and Alex

December 14, 2007

What started off as a tough week has turned into a much better one. By Day 2 of Taylor's steroids, her demeanor was just impossible. We know it is hard on her, but it is also so hard on those around her too. You can only tell yourself so many times 'It's the medicine,' but it truly is. For some reason, the steroids seem to hit her system much quicker now, but the 'bad' effects (i.e., the really bad attitude) also seem to only last through the end of Day 3. On Day 4 and 5, she still had an increased appetite, but overall everything was manageable. It gets really hard sometimes- just so frustrating, but you just continue to tell yourself that this has a purpose, and that eventually, we will get through this. I am so thankful for the offers of help- including Grandma, Grandpa and Aunt Debbie who just showed up on Sunday and said "Give us one of the girls- we'll divide and conquer- it is too much with the 2 of them right now." With Rob on shift that day, I was so appreciative, and then each of the girls got the attention they needed at that time. It also cut down on the fighting between the 2 of them over toys, etc....which on steroids gets just ridiculous!

All of that said, the week has turned out fine. We made trips to see the Living Nativity here in town last weekend, and Taylor and Alex both just loved it. Taylor went back a second time with her Daddy on Sunday night. She loves hearing the story about the night Baby Jesus was born. I think I've told her that story every night this week before bedtime.

We have a weekend of baking cookies as well as plans of seeing 'The Nutcracker.' I think it will be a really nice weekend. I hope everyone is having a good holiday season. I think that everything seems magnified to us this year- or maybe we are just taking a little more time to soak it all in. Either way, we are just enjoying watching the kids take it all in. Take care, and we will keep everyone posted on her progress.

Love, Rob, Kim, Taylor, and Alex

December 27, 2007

We hope everyone had a wonderful Christmas. Things here were great! We had a busy week, filled with a trip to Port Saint Lucie to visit with Rob's family and then back to Tallahassee for Christmas Eve and Christmas Day activities at home and at Grandma and Grandpa's house. Although it was busy traveling back and forth, it was great to see family, and Santa managed to stop at 3 houses for the girls! He was just chasing them around Florida! Leading up to Christmas, I prayed each day that Taylor would continue to stay healthy and be able to spend Christmas at home. When Christmas morning came, and she woke up in her own bed, it was truly a blessing.

Prior to heading out of town to Port Saint Lucie, we also had Taylor's counts checked. Her counts have remained strong (ANC was over 1,000), and it was a comfortable checkpoint for us before we hit the road. She has a 2 day visit to Gainesville next week for her monthly chemotherapy as well as her lumbar puncture (the spinal chemotherapy she receives every 3 months). Things continue to progress, yet there are still days you wonder how you got here. One thing that continues to amaze me is Taylor's strength. I know that she doesn't understand the gravity of everything going on, but she is just so much wiser than she needs to be for a 4 year old....and having to consider things that her friends don't necessarily have to deal with. Sometimes, these stories can be sweet though....like on Christmas morning: Taylor came downstairs and ran to the table to see if Santa had eaten his cookies. Sure enough, there were lots of crumbs, but still one cookie left. She asked if she could have it, and I said "Sure sweetie, I'm sure Santa left it for you." She picked it up, and then put it down and said "Mommy, what if Santa has germs? I'm not supposed to share food...." I told her that I'm sure he knew she was going to eat that cookie, and that he purposely didn't touch it. She was okay with that.

Christmas is also just such a reflective time. On Christmas Eve, I was reading the girls their bedtime books, and Taylor's book was about the night that Jesus was born. She asked me if she would get to meet Jesus when she went to heaven, and I told her that we all do. She told me that she didn't want to go to heaven by herself, and that she didn't want to go there without me, Daddy, and Alex...and I told her that everything would be okay, and that none of us are going anywhere anytime soon. I have to admit that I choked back some tears on that one, but at the same time- there is such a refreshing innocence on her perspective about things, and I want her to feel comforted that everything is okay....enough teary stories though- all in all, everything is going just great! And we couldn't have asked for a better Christmas this year. We were just so happy to all be together.

We have some adorable pictures of the girls from this past week, and I promise to upload them...as soon as I troubleshoot whatever issue I'm having with uploading them from the camera this morning. So....maybe some pictures later this week!

Love to all, and have a very Happy New Year!

Love, Rob, Kim, Taylor, and Alex

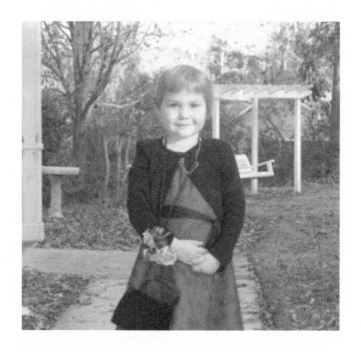

2008

Happy New Year! (Yes, I know...we are already 1 week into the New Year, but it has been a busy week...lots to update!)

Taylor had a busy 2 day trip to Gainesville this week, including her clinic visit on Thursday and her lumbar puncture procedure on Friday (the spinal chemo she receives every 3 months during the Maintenance phase). Because her treatment fell over the holidays, we decided to head down a day early on Wednesday and drive to Orlando for a day trip to Downtown Disney. It was a good time (but really cold!), so I was happy that we had not made plans to go to the parks or do anything that required us to stay outside for an extended period of time....Thursday morning, we headed over to a character breakfast at Chef Mickey's so that the girls could see their favorite characters from Mickey Mouse Clubhouse...and then it was off to Gainesville for a clinic visit. Many thanks to Grandma who made the trip with us, and helped out tremendously with the girls.

Taylor's counts were up (ANC over 1900), so her doctors decided to resume her daily chemo to a full dosage. This means her full dose of 6-MP every night, and she is bumped back up to 6 pills of Methotrexate every Friday night. We also started her 5 day stint of steroids (which I am happy to say we are 2 days from being through!), so it has been an emotional weekend as well. Overall, she has handled the steroids a little better this time around, but there are still times where the littlest things have set her off. We are making it through though, and we just remind ourselves that this is part of the regimen...

I've uploaded some pictures from Christmas and the New Year...and of course some pictures from Disney. The girls have had a busy couple of weeks, but there are lots of good memories. Taylor stayed up to watch the ball drop on New Year's Eve (I could hardly keep my eyes open!), but she made a resolution to 'be nice to her little sister.' We think she already does a good job of being a protective big sis, but any thought of being even a little nicer to your sibling can't be a bad thing, so we told her we were very proud of her.

We are hopeful that 2008 continues to bring good news for Taylor, and for everyone out there who is having to fight this awful disease. As I sat in the waiting room at the hospital on Friday, I had flash backs to January 2007 when I was waiting in that same room with Rob, Alex, my sister, and parents-wondering if the doctors were going to come out of the biopsy and confirm that Taylor truly did have cancer. The time we spent waiting was torture, but then once you know- you just act. You just take it all day by day. Please pray for those who are waiting on test results or who are newly diagnosed and trying to understand the direction this is going to take them and their families. Sometimes the waiting, and the 'not knowing' can be the hardest part.

Lastly, I'd ask that everyone keep Rob's mom in your prayers. She was admitted to the hospital this weekend, and we are awaiting feedback from her doctors as to how long she will have to stay there.

To end on a happy note, we do wish everyone a very happy and healthy 2008, and I will keep everyone posted on Taylor's progress. She will have her counts checked here locally next week (to monitor the increased chemo dosage and any impacts to her counts). We'll let you know how it goes!

Love, Rob, Kim, Taylor, and Alex

January 18, 2008

The past few days have stirred up quite a few memories from a year ago. It was 1 year ago today that Taylor's school called Rob and I to tell us that she fell asleep during 'circle time' and that she was running a fever of 102 degrees.....So, I go to pick her up, figuring we're home for a day or so on some Tylenol, and you move on. Wow, was I wrong!

This weekend, January 20th, will be the 1 year mark for Taylor (in terms of the official biopsy and diagnosis). We've learned so much in the past year, in addition to my crash course in medical terminology. Most importantly I think we've learned that above all, you have to have faith and know that there is a bigger plan. No one is ever going to think it's 'fair' that a child gets cancer and has to endure everything that she has in the past year, and for the next 15 months. Unless you succumb to the idea that there was a bigger purpose for all of this, you would never get through it (sane anyway).

Carson (the little boy from Tallahassee that was diagnosed just a couple of days prior to Taylor) is at the year mark as well, and his mom put everything in such an amazing way (www.caringbridge.org/visit/carsonchapman). Her last point was amazing- because while it's true- you wouldn't wish this on anyone- we appreciate that God has given us each other to go through this together.

And God gave us all of you to support us through this. We can't say enough thank yous

- to our family and friends who were there to give Alex the attention and care she needed, and continue to be there to help throughout this whole process

- to our employers who were flexible with our schedules and essentially let us 'check out' for whatever time we needed to

- to everyone who donated hours at work so that we could take the time off we needed with Taylor, and not miss a paycheck

- to those who sent cards, toys, snacks, dinners, gas cards, restaurant gift cards- everything was so appreciated

- and to everyone who checks in on this website to follow Taylor's progress....this website has been a blessing for us to keep everyone updated.

We will be forever grateful.

On a more recent note, Taylor had her counts checked this week at KidsKorner. She has been on her full dose of chemo for a 2-week period now, and her ANC has held at 990. Her white blood cell count, platelets, hematocrit and hemoglobin were all at good levels too, so we will continue to hope that her body handles the chemo well (at this resumed level).

Well, I'll sign off for now, but please know how much your thoughtfulness and prayers have gotten us through the past year. Love to all, and believe me- there will be a heck of a party when we get to March 22, 2009....love, Rob, Kim, Taylor, and Alex

January 20, 2008

Thank you to everyone for your postings this week. When I've talked to so many of you this week....I know you also say that it is hard to believe that it's been a year.....that made me think that it might be good to post some pictures from this past year, so I took some time to do that this morning.

We are spending time with Grandma and Aunt Debbie this morning, and then heading to the fire station to visit Daddy....so I'll make this entry short. Love to all, and we'll keep you posted on Taylor's progress this week.

Love, Rob, Kim, Taylor, and Alex

January 25, 2008

What an exciting week for Taylor! The Dreams Come True foundation called us last week (the foundation that sent her to California for the 'Dancing with the Stars' rehearsal), and let us know that they had set aside 3 tickets for the 'Dancing with the Stars' tour for us if we would like to take Taylor. I was so appreciative that they continue to think of Taylor, and she was so excited when I picked her up from school that day and told her the news!

So, off we went to Jacksonville this past Tuesday night. I'll admit that a Tuesday night show 2+ hours away kinda scared me (in terms of thinking about school the next day!)- but we were absolutely going. We just packed some PJs in the car for her, and she slept all the way home after the show. She looked like a little princess in her pretty red dress (and silver crown she picked out to wear). It brought back a lot of great memories from our trip in October. One of the most memorable parts of the night was when we had a chance to stand in line to meet one of the dancers (Mark- Sabrina's dance partner from this past season). When we got to the front of the line, and had a chance to talk with him, I started off by saying "Hi Mark, I'm not sure if you remember, but we had a chance to meet you when we came out to a rehearsal...." Before I could finish, he said "I do remember her- you were at a rehearsal, and she had her pretty dress on..." Long story short, he truly did remember Miss Taylor spinning around on the dance floor back in October. I told him that it truly meant a lot that he remembered her visit to the show....and of course, it just endeared me to the cast of that show even more! What amazing folks!!!

So, she had an exciting evening out on Tuesday. Many thanks to Grandpa and Aunt Debbie who kept Alex and had a 'special date' to go to dinner and play. Grandma made the trip with Taylor and me (and looked like she enjoyed the show as well!). Taylor can't wait to show her Daddy her pretty dress. He has been in South Florida spending time with Gammy (Rob's mom), and hoping that she will be able to leave the hospital soon. We continue to keep her in our prayers.

The rest of the week went well for Taylor. We took a trip to KidsKorner to get her counts checked, as I was concerned that she was looking a little pale and sounding stuffy. Turned out that her counts had maintained at over 940. This was really amazing to me, as she has now been on her 100% dose of daily and weekly chemo for 3 weeks now. She is stronger than she even knows! Her white blood cell count, hematocrit and hemoglobin, and platelets were all at acceptable levels too. She just continues to amaze us.

She'll have a trip to Gainesville next week for her IV chemo, and a check-up with the doctors. We'll keep everyone posted, and thank you again for checking in on Miss Taylor. Love to all....

Love, Rob, Kim, Taylor and Alex.

February 4, 2008

I'll start with the good news! Taylor had a productive visit to clinic last Thursday, with an ANC of over 1,000. We continue to be amazed at the strength of her little body, and how it is maintaining acceptable count levels at her full dosage of chemotherapy. With good counts, it also made us feel comfortable about her big 'date night' with Daddy this past Saturday night. Taylor and Daddy went to the Daddy / Daughter dance this weekend, along with some of her friends from the neighborhood, and her very first friend

(Madison). Madison and Taylor were born an hour apart, and their Daddy's work together at the fire department.... The Daddy's decided to surprise the girls with a limo for the dance. You can imagine the look on 5 little faces when the car pulled up- and they found out there was a DVD player to play a Hannah Montana movie. It was really fun to see how excited they were. Rob got Taylor a corsage, and she spent half the day getting ready for her date. They had a blast.

Rob said that Taylor behaved really well, which was a relief to both of us- as we didn't originally notice that the dance coincided with Day 2 of her monthly steroid stint. Her steroid side effects didn't seem to kick in bad until Sunday, and then today has just been crazy. It started off okay, but then by breakfast time, she was in such an outrage that she was throwing stuff out of the pantry in frustration. She couldn't find what she wanted to eat, and when she finally did- it was 8 am and time to get to school. I explained to her that she could not have chicken soup as there wasn't time to make it, but that just elevated the outburst. It's not good for Alex to see Taylor so outraged (as it scares her), so I got Alex's things packed up in the car, and set her up in her car seat with a snack while I tried to calm Taylor down. Within a couple of minutes, I had Taylor outside, but she was screaming at the top of her lungs. She cried all the way to school, and refused to go inside. She continued to try and find anything in the car to throw to get my attention. On top of everything, she truly is fighting a cough (no temperature thankfully), but she just kept crying that she needed to go home because she was sick. Finally, I figured I needed to just throw in the towel for the day- so I called into work, and was appreciative that they understood. One of the teachers took Alex inside, and I headed home with Taylor. After beating myself up on the way home over everything and how I could have maybe done something different...I reminded myself that this is the 1st time we've had to keep her home during a steroid stint. So overall, we should be thankful that she continues to handle everything okay. I called Rob at the fire station, and he re-minded me of the same thing- and then reminded me of the more important thing- that it is a year later, and she is still with us.

So with that perspective, she and I are trying to make the most of our day together. She is on a little bit of an eating binge at the moment....ham, pickles, Rice Krispies and Chicken Soup....so I told her we are going to leave the house in a bit to get some fresh air. Hopefully that will get her mind off of eating.

She told me that she is going to school tomorrow because she is sure that they are learning about something very important. I also made her promise that to Miss Kylie (her teacher) this morning when we saw her at school.

Overall though, I have to remember we still have awhile to go on this journey....I am going to start a steroid countdown though. After she wraps up her stint tomorrow, there will only be 13 months left of steroids. Yea!!!!

Thank you for everyone's notes, and we will keep you posted on her progress this week. Love to all....

Love, Rob, Kim, Taylor, and Alex

February 10, 2008

As I write this update, I have just finished a new webpage...'Team Princess Taylor's' Relay for Life site (http://main.acsevents.org/goto/teamprincesstaylor).

Friends, family and coworkers had 2 teams for Taylor last year at the Relay for Life, and Rob and I were so appreciative. This year, we are honored to take on the responsibility of coordinating the team and doing fundraising activities. Taylor went to the team captain meeting with me this past Thursday night, and she could not stop talking about it on the way home. She is even putting extra change in her Relay for Life piggybank for donations.

The event is April 11th - 12th, and we would love everyone to come out and walk, so if you are interested- click on the link above and join Taylor's team! I think it is an amazing event (very emotional as you can imagine), and it brings together so many people that have been touched by this disease....whether you are a survivor, caregiver, or a concerned family member / friend...it is an unforgettable experience. Drop me an e-mail at kakoegel@comcast.net if you want to chat further about it, but Rob and I look forward to a good turnout and good time with family and friends.

Taylor's week improved- slowly but surely. The side effects from steroids are something that I don't wish on anyone- but it is what it is...they help her maintain the strength she needs to fight this disease. She is so strong, and as I said on my 'Team Princess Taylor' page tonight- as a four year old- she has taught me more about life and living in the past year than most adults I know.

Love to all, and we will keep you posted on her progress this week. She will have her counts checked here locally, and we are hopeful that her body continues to maintain acceptable count levels...

Love, Rob, Kim, Taylor, and Alex

February 15, 2008

Hope everyone had a nice Valentine's Day! Taylor and Alex had a wonderful surprise last night- when a 'singing Valentine' arrived at our door! Many thanks to our neighbors who arranged for a singing quartet for the girls- it truly was an amazing and thoughtful gift. Among other songs, they sang 'Let me call you sweetheart' to the girls. Each of the girls also received a red carnation, and Mommy received a box of chocolates....these gentlemen are part of a group called the 'Capital Chordsmen.' It was such a neat gift, and they were extremely talented!

Taylor had her counts checked at KidsKorner on Wednesday, and we received great news that she continues to maintain acceptable count levels at the 100% dosage of chemo. Her overall ANC was 1200, and her hemoglobin, hematocrit, and platelets were at good levels too. I know I sound like a broken record sometimes, but the strength of her little body continues to amaze me.

She is fighting a cough (that seems to come from her toes!) It does concern me, and we are just keeping a close eye on her- any threat of illness is cause for concern. We can just take it day by day though, and be thankful that otherwise everything is fine. She has good energy, a good appetite, and is very happy right now.

Well, I am off to work- so love to everyone, and thank you

again for following Taylor's site. Before I sign off, I just want to thank everyone for the support for Taylor's Relay for Life team too. We would love for you to come walk with us....it is an amazing event. If you get a chance, check out her 'Team Princess Taylor' Relay for Life site (http://main.ac-sevents.org/goto/teamprincesstaylor).

Have a great weekend, and we will keep you posted. Love, Rob, Kim, Taylor, and Alex

February 18, 2008

A busy day- but a good result. Taylor had the cough that wouldn't quit, and we were beginning to get concerned. Even though she's been a bundle of energy, been in a good mood, and had a good appetite...it still worried me. And then this morning, she ran a fever that hit 100.3 degrees. So...it was time to call Shands and her local pediatrician to understand what we should do. Still a bundle of energy, she and I headed to the pediatrician's office this morning and then to Kids Korner for labs and a subsequent chest

x-ray. The good news: the x-ray came back negative (i.e., no sign of pneumonia or any concerns in her chest), and her counts were high. They may have been high because her white blood cell count was up (meaning her body is possibly fighting an infection), so her doctors prescribed an IV anti-biotic just to cover for that. She enjoyed her time at the hospital, as she got to paint a ceiling tile while she received her medicine....The child life specialist at TMH(Miss Michelle) is so wonderful to the kids there, and had told Taylor that she could paint a tile today.....so Taylor was thrilled.

She didn't skip a beat today, and she maintained a good level of energy throughout the rest of the day....but her daddy and I were extremely relieved. There will continue to be scares, but we will just try to get through each one and move on. Today turned out just fine (although we're pretty tired!)

And continued thank yous to the folks who have signed up

for the 'Team Princess Taylor' Relay for Life team. You can check out the team site at http://main.acsevents.org/goto/ teamprincesstaylor.

We'll keep everyone posted, as Taylor will head to Gainesville for a checkup next week. Thank you again for your prayers. They continue to get us through this journey. Love, Rob, Kim, Taylor, and Alex

February 26, 2008

I love this picture of Taylor and Kody. She and Kody have known each other since they were 3 months old (and at home daycare together at Granny's house!) They are still in school together, and were dance partners for their Fairytale Ball last Friday. Taylor talked about it for a month, and the kids practiced so hard! She got a little nervous when she came out and saw the crowd of parents waiting to see them dance, and she missed 'her spin,' which she was a little upset about (in fact, she wanted me to call Kody's mommy and have her drive him over to our house so that they could spin again)- but she has

now calmed down about all of that. She was just so excited to get all dressed up in her pretty pink dress- it was really a neat event for the kids.

She continued with her busy weekend and headed to her friend Graham's birthday party on Saturday. The kids had a blast (as it was at a horse farm), and I just wish I had the pictures to upload....I was having a technical issue with my camera this morning- but I'll figure that out! I was so proud of both of the girls, as they rode the horses several times, and had a good time playing with friends.

Taylor is continuing on her antibiotics for a couple more days (from last Monday's visit to the doctor), but they have helped tremendously. The yucky cough is barely there, and she has seemed to feel well overall. She makes a trip to Shands this week for her monthly check-up, so we feel good about her doctors seeing her too. She has had a little bit of an attitude lately, but again- we are not sure how much of it is being 4 and how much of it is due to frustration about treatment, acting out, etc. We'd like to continue that discussion with her doctors as well. I asked her the other day "Taylor, why are you yelling and screaming?" and she told me "It's my medicine." I asked her which one, and she told me "It's my Methotrexate." I told her that her Methotrexate does not make her do that, and that she needs to learn to control herself a little better. That seemed to fall on deaf ears....so I told her "If you continue to act up, there is no Disney Channel"- that seemed to have more of an impact. We'll see what happens.

Well, we'll keep everyone posted on her week and her trip to Shands. Team Princess Taylor (http://main.acsevents.org/goto/teamprincesstaylor) continues to do awesome! The team has raised over $1,000 to date for the Relay for Life- so thank you to everyone who has made that happen. Your support is very appreciated.

Take care, and have a great week. Love, Rob, Kim, Taylor, and Alex

March 2, 2008

Taylor's trip to Gainesville went great this week. Her ANC was at 1575, which is higher than it normally is, but it's been an interesting couple of weeks between her various antibiotics and the cough / cold she was fighting off...The remainder of her counts (her platelets, hematocrit and hemoglobin) were at good levels too, so it was just a standard visit (i.e., she received her IV chemo, saw her doctors, and made it back within a 1 day visit). She is on Day 3 of steroids, and it comes with its ups and downs, but as of this morning's dose- we are 50% through! So, we just take it in chunks. Many thanks to Grandma and Grandpa who helped to divide and conquer yesterday and spent the day with Alex. That one on one time gives her so much attention, and it's just wonderful.

Taylor had a busy week, filled with Grandpa's birthday (and cupcakes and ice cream cake), Graham's birthday party (with lots of horsey rides!), and a pizza night with friends on Friday night. The daddy's watched the kids and gave the moms a night out at the Keith Urban / Carrie Underwood concert on Friday night. It was a fun night out with the girls- which all of us need once in a while! Although, I did lose it when Carrie Underwood sang "Jesus take the wheel...." It's just such a beautiful song, and I guess that's just how things feel sometimes....

Rob reminded me last night that she only has 12 more visits to Shands before her end of treatment date. When he said it like that, it feels like it is within reach. He has an amazing way of keeping me sane through all of this!

Thanks again to everyone's support of Team Princess Taylor (http://main.acsevents.org/goto/teamprincesstaylor). The team has raised over $1,700 to date for the Relay for Life- so thank you to everyone who has made that happen. There's still a few days to sign up if you want to walk with us! The deadline is March 5th (in order for them to have t-shirts ready for the team), so think about it, and sign up if you'd like to walk on our team! We'd love to have you.

Take care, and have a great week. Love, Rob, Kim, Taylor, and Alex

March 3, 2008

I just had to take a picture of these wonderful chocolate ribbons from Miss Kathryn. A surprise package arrived in the mail this weekend with these chocolate 'Leukemia awareness' ribbons (I know you are wondering- so I will tell you what they taste like. They are white chocolate with orange coloring- and yes they are delicious!)

They come complete with a sticker on the back with the 'Team Princess Taylor' website (http://main.acsevents.org/goto/teamprincesstaylor) and Kathryn had the great idea of selling them at the tent the night of the 'Relay for Life' as our tent fundraiser. Thank you so much! I know I've told her a million times, but I'll say it again- she is an amazing lady, and she and her family have been so thoughtful throughout this whole process....Germy still sits on Taylor's dresser and watches over her at night (and eats up all of the yucky germs that might even try to come close to Taylor).

Everyone will hear us cheering tomorrow night when we are done with the 5 day steroid stint! Only 12 more stints to go! (Yesterday I thought it was 11, but I think I counted wrong)- but 12 is within reach! Overall, she has done well this time around, but she has had her moments. She hasn't been sleeping very soundly (the steroids just never seem to allow very restful sleep), but she finally drifted off a few minutes ago. The doctors gave us instructions about giving Benadryl to help her sleep when she is on her steroid stint, but even that doesn't seem to help consistently. Your heart just breaks for her, because you know she is tired, but her little body can't completely relax. Tonight, it seemed to work- so that is good. Hopefully she will get a good night's rest. I let her come downstairs to watch Hannah Montana after Alex went to bed, so she is sleeping right next to me as I type this. I'll probably give it a few minutes before carrying her upstairs....I want to make sure she is REALLY sleeping...

Thank you again for your prayers and postings. And I wanted to tell you about an amazing little girl who is so close to the end of her treatment for the same cancer. Miss Samantha Lee (www.caringbridge.org/visit/samanthalee) is a little over a month away. What a fighter she is! I have followed her site religiously over the past year, and have learned a lot from her and her family....there is definitely a virtual support group in the midst of all of this!

Have a good week, and we'll keep you posted on Taylor's progress. Love, Rob, Kim, Taylor, and Alex

March 6, 2008

Today was a great day. In fact, it was Taylor's 'special day' at school, and she was looking forward to it all week. Each student in her class is assigned a 'special day' where he/she gets to bring in a treat for the class, be the line leader, sit in a special seat during circle time, etc.

She has been talking about her 'special day' all week, and honestly, it must have been like a light at the end of the tunnel for her this week (especially coming off of steroids). She bounced out of bed this morning and got dressed in record time (in a beautiful party dress for her 'special day'), and she decided she wanted to bring in 3 versions of Rice Krispie treats today. She asked me to make plain ones, ones with sprinkles, and ones with chocolate frosting on top. Needless to say, I had my share of sugar last night getting those ready. It was definitely worth it though- seeing how excited she was about everything today.

She's still having a little bit of trouble totally relaxing at night and being able to go to sleep at a normal time (i.e., she's sitting next to me watching Hannah Montana as I type), but that's okay. You can already see a marked difference in her appetite and her demeanor. It's been a great day...

Today was a great day for another reason too. Taylor's uncle who has been going through a battle with cancer germs received good news today that the cancer was encapsulated (I think I spelled that right, but it means that the cancer was contained to the part that was removed during his surgery). It was a relief to hear that wonderful news, and an answered prayer.

We're continuing to get ready for the Relay for Life (http://main.acsevents.org/goto/teamprincesstaylor), as it will be here before we know it! Thank you to everyone- Team Princess Taylor is very close to their goal!

We'll keep you posted on Taylor's progress this week. She'll make a trip to KidsKorner next week for her midpoint check on her counts. We'll have to check out if the 'Rainbow Rock' tile is hanging up! Have a great week.

Love, Rob, Kim, Taylor, and Alex

March 17, 2008

Happy St. Patrick's Day! Taylor and Alex should be up shortly, and already have their 'green' clothes ready to go. Although- for any of you who have heard me talk about Alex's fashion sense, she may want to change her outfit 20 or 30 times this morning before we head out the door....I have to remember to laugh about it or I'd go crazy!

Taylor seems to be feeling good overall. She complains of nausea more now than she did before; however, she seems able to get past it and get on with her day. Sometimes I have to stop and remember that this child is on daily doses of chemo. To think that she would never feel sick to her stomach is unrealistic. It is odd though how mechanical a lot of this becomes- administering medicine, etc. Her demeanor has varied- we'll have a great 3 or 4 days, and then there will be lots of attitude. It is tiring and very trying, but in my mind, every dose brings us closer to her end of treatment date. It is just a little over 1 year away.

It has been a good and busy couple of weeks for the girls. Their time has been filled with Easter egg hunts, birthday parties, and spending time with Grandma, Grandpa and Aunt Debbie. Grandpa is in Egypt right now for work (which Taylor is very excited about, because she knows where Africa is on the globe....and she is hoping Grandpa sees a camel while he is there). Grandpa won't be home in time for Easter, so we had a special Easter dinner for him at Carrabas before he left.

The girls are excited about Easter, and it is interesting to me how Taylor is very focused on the true meaning of the holiday. She very clearly remembers the children's' sermon from last Easter at Bee Ridge (our church in Sarasota)...when Pastor Karl put rocks on top of a cardboard box (to simulate the stone in front of Jesus' tomb). When he took the rocks off, helium balloons rose out of the box and to the top of the church. Taylor reminded me last night at church that when we go to heaven, we live again- just like Jesus. I try to treasure her perspective on things like this- it is just so pure, and it reminds me that even though she is 4, she is trying to process all of these concepts!

The Relay for Life preparation continues for Team Princess Taylor(http://main.acsevents.org/goto/teamprincesstaylor). We had a team drop- in last weekend to start coordinating some of the logistics for the event, but mostly for the team members to meet and just socialize. Taylor attended a team captain meeting with me last week, and her team is top of the list for online fundraising, so thank you to everyone who is supporting her.

She will head to Gainesville next week for her monthly check-up, chemo, and her quarterly lumbar puncture. We just continue to pray that all of this turns out okay for Taylor. I have to remind myself that God already has a plan. Of course, selfishly, I am just hoping that his plan is the same as ours is for Taylor. She is such a strong little girl, as are all of the kids fighting childhood cancer. Thank you for your continued prayers and support. We'll keep you posted on her progress! Love, Rob, Kim, Taylor, and Alex

March 18, 2008

Miss Taylor rushed home from ballet class tonight- as soon as she remembered that 'Dancing with the Stars' was on again...I have never seen her get a bath and pajamas on so quickly. She was very sweet, as she wanted to help get Alex to bed first and then she put a Cinderella gown on over her pajamas (She said she didn't want Alex to feel left out, so she wanted to wait until Alex was asleep to put the Cinderella gown on). So, she had a special night and got a chance to stay up a little late to watch the show. We are recording all of them anyway, so I'm sure the episodes will be on non-stop regardless.

It's a little early for her to pick her favorites, but she definitely liked Priscilla and Marissa tonight. She especially liked Miss Marissa's 'Apple Bottom' jeans song...but she was also amazed that Miss Marlee (Marlee Matlin) was able to dance even though she can't hear the music. I told her that it takes a special person to be brave enough to try things that nobody else thinks they can do. Taylor thought she should have gotten a '10' because she did so well. I have to agree...

Taylor had a good day today- a little bit of a rough start to the week yesterday, as she woke up with a lot of nausea. After some ginger ale, she perked up, but she was insistent about not feeling well enough to go to school. She didn't have a temperature, and her appetite started to come back, so I went with my gut and took her to school (knowing that there is still a long road, and while I wish she could stay home every time she doesn't feel well, that is just not realistic). So, with no temp, we headed off to school. Many thanks to her teachers and the staff at Scottsdale who helped to calm her down and held her when I left. She ended up having a great day at school, and told us all about the leprechaun that visited her classroom while they were outside (her teachers are so creative).

So, on with the rest of the week! We'll keep you posted on her progress, including her trip to Gainesville next week. Love to all....Love, Rob, Kim, Taylor, and Alex

March 24, 2008

Hope everyone had a nice Easter! This past weekend was a busy and fun weekend, and most importantly- the beginning of the 'countdown' to the end of treatment. As of Saturday, March 22nd, Taylor is 1 year away from her end of chemotherapy. I considered getting a 'countdown clock,' and then Rob and I remembered that even when the chemo is done- the worry won't stop. While it will be a huge milestone, there will always be concern; however, I'm sure that will ease over time. Regardless, we can see the light at the end of the tunnel for her daily, weekly, monthly, and quarterly chemo-therapy, and we continue to just be so proud of her and her strength throughout this.

She made us proud on so many levels this weekend, including her first skate party for a friend at school. Even though she took her share of spills, she was determined to skate around the rink with her friends this weekend. She had an amazing time, and wants to go back again. I told her we'd go for les-sons on Saturdays if she'd like....and she told me she wants Mommy to put some skates on too. I told her it's been awhile (so I'm hoping that it's like riding a bike!) We'll see...

One adorable thing about this weekend (in addition to the egg hunt, Easter morning, dying eggs, etc.)- she caught part of the 'Ten Commandments' on Saturday night before she went to bed. She was excited to see that Moses was in Egypt, and was hoping that he would run into Grandpa while he was there. She kept on asking "When is Moses going to see Grandpa? Is he at the pyramids?"

She woke up this morning and must have had a sense that this is her clinic / lumbar puncture week at Shands. She in-formed me that she is canceling her next trip to clinic and that I should call Shands to tell them so, and that she would reschedule for Sunday. Not sure why there is the heightened sensitivity (i.e., meaning more than normal), or why there is a preference for Sunday- but I told her I would call clinic to see if they are open on Sunday. She said if they aren't open, then she will go on Thursday. I told her that is a deal.....so, she and Daddy will head to Gainesville for her Vincristine (the IV chemo) and her lumbar puncture (the spinal chemo) later this week.

We'll keep everyone posted on her progress this week. Please keep her in your prayers as she undergoes her treatments this week. And thank you again to everyone's support of Team Princess Taylor (http://main.acsevents.org/goto/teamprin-cesstaylor). The Relay is almost here! And Taylor informed me she is bringing her baby stroller to push her dolls around the track with her.

Take care, and we'll post more later this week. Love, Rob, Kim, Taylor, and Alex

March 27, 2008

I just talked to Rob, and Taylor is sleeping soundly....a good end to a long day that started off with lots of yelling and screaming about not wanting to go to clinic.

While it has been a topic of conversation all week, Taylor was pretty adamant last night and this morning about not going to Gainesville. I can imagine that getting IV and spinal chemo is not fun by any means, but I can't remember a time in the past 6 months that she has been this anxious about a trip to Shands. Thankfully, Rob was able to pick her up from school without a big scene...and they made their way to Gainesville. Her checkup went well, with an ANC over 1200. Her platelets, hematocrit, and hemoglobin were all at acceptable levels too. She woke up with a cough this morning, but her doctors didn't seem concerned- just said to keep an eye on it. She'll have her lumbar puncture in the morning (the spinal chemo), and then head home to Tallahassee with Daddy.

One issue that Rob talked to her doctors about was the increase in nausea / vomiting in the mornings. It has gotten increasingly worse over the past couple of months. Typically, after some ginger ale and little bites of food, she's able to get past it, but it is awful to watch her go through this in the morning. Rob and I were wondering if it had something to do with low blood sugar in the morning (and the fact that by that point she has typically gone 12 - 13 hours without any food due to having to eat dinner so early for her Nighttime chemo). Her doctors mentioned having something small to eat prior to bedtime (which surprised us as the original direction was to take the medicine on an empty stomach and as close to bedtime as possible). They explained that if she waits at least an hour after the medicine, but has something small, it should be okay. We'll see how she does, as this will be a balance of not encouraging too much to eat but making sure she has enough in her body to balance out her blood sugars. We'll get through it, and figure out what's best, but it is definitely a learning experience.

Taylor's steroid stint starts tomorrow, and I get anxious just thinking about it. I know that we just have to take it day by day. It is hard perspective to keep sometimes, especially in the midst of an eating binge or an anger rage. I just try to be thankful that Rob and I have each other as well as a wonderful network of support. And sometimes you just need a good cry. I find that works well too.

Ironically, as I type this, I just saw an interview about a new book by Dr. Laura called "Stop Whining, and Start Living." I think I may pick that up this weekend. Supposedly it discusses how people focus so much on the past or worry about the future that they forget to focus on the amazing things going on around them right now. While I feel like I've gained a ton of perspective in the past year, it still seems like a good message to read. I definitely still focus on times before Taylor got sick or worry about scenarios of relapse, etc....and it is important to put those thoughts to the side. We'll see- if I can find a few minutes to give it a read, I'll let you know how it goes!

We'll keep everyone posted on her progress this week. Please also keep Carson Chapman in your prayers (www.caringbridge.org/visit/carsonchapman). He has been admitted to the hospital as a result of the flu, and is going stir crazy at the moment (understandably!). Hopefully his counts will start to come up and he can come home soon.

Take care, and we'll post more later this week.

Love, Rob, Kim, Taylor, and Alex

April 10, 2008

It's been a busy week as we look ahead to the American Cancer Society 'Relay for Life' this Friday night. Taylor was up drawing pictures tonight to 'decorate the tent.' She also decorated a luminaria bag, and is anticipating getting to walk around the track with family and friends this coming weekend. It's an emotional event, and a constant reminder of the events of the past 15 months, but I am happy that we are able to participate. Team Princess Taylor has nearly doubled its original fundraising goal, so thank you to everyone who has helped make that happen.(http://main.acsevents.org/goto/teamprincesstaylor).

It's been an interesting couple of weeks- some ups and downs. Taylor's nausea in the mornings continues, making us think that there may be concerns with her blood sugar levels (as she is nauseous and then after some juice, ginger ale, small bits of food, etc.- she'll start to perk up). Additionally, her moods can be erratic in the morning- so then we think there may be times when her sugar is too high. Typically once she gets some food into her, things seem to settle down-sometimes the attitude continues- it's challenging. We are going to just continue the conversations with her doctors. Our understanding from them is that the combination of the steroids and the chemotherapy regimen can cause diabetes (or at a minimum blood sugar challenges) during treatment-so we just want to make sure we are addressing. It's just hard-and you don't know what the morning is going to bring for her or how she is going to feel. We just know that we have to persevere, and get through the next 11 months of chemotherapy.

We made a trip down to Sarasota with Grandma and Grandpa this weekend. I'll apologize now for not being able to drop in and see some friends while we were in town, but it was a pretty quick trip, and it was a pretty packed couple of days. We were so happy to get to spend some time with Aunt Florence and Uncle Lou (my great aunt and uncle). Uncle Lou is turning 90 today! Happy Birthday! We also got to spend time with Aunt Carol, Uncle Buddy, and Kelly, and had the chance to see our Bee Ridge family at church on Sunday- and the girls are in love with Siesta Beach- so we definitely made a stop there. They played hard, and ran back and forth from the waves for a good 2 hours. There were good naps following the beach (yea!!!) Taylor and Alex look so happy in the pictures from the beach. It's times like those that help you get through some of the yucky times- knowing that there are still times when both of them can still just be normal little kids (I constantly remind myself that Alex is just as impacted by all of this- not all 2 year old's are having to deal with the side effects of a sibling in treatment...she's gonna be a tough kid too!)

Taylor had ballet on Tuesday night, and her recital outfit arrived (so she is very excited- and has tried it on at least 5 times already!) It was interesting because the outfit came with a hair ribbon to wrap around a bun in her hair. She looked at me kind of funny about that when her teacher was explaining it, and I promised Taylor after class that if she wanted me to clip it into her hair somehow- we'd figure it out! All in all, she didn't seem overly concerned about it, and in all honesty- I'm not quite sure how to make a fancy bun in her hair anyway, so we'll play it all by ear and see if she even cares about it when it's time for the recital next month. It's all perspective.

Some exciting news- Taylor is going to have the chance to head out to California for another 'Dancing with the Stars' rehearsal over the next couple of weeks...she is excited, (although sad to see Miss Julianne voted off the show last night). Thank you to Grandpa for offering up his frequent flier miles for the trip. We'll post some pictures, and are just again appreciative to ABC and Dancing with the Stars for their offer for her to come to another rehearsal. I can't even explain how much she looks forward to that show. Lord knows- it got us through a good bit of her early treatments with having to stay up late for her medicine. It was such a distraction for her from all of the bad stuff going on- and she would dance around the house for the 2 hours it was on each night.

Hope everyone is doing well, and we will keep you posted on her progress this week. Love, Rob, Kim, Taylor, and Alex

April 15, 2008

What a busy weekend! The Relay for Life was Friday night through Saturday morning....and Team Princess Taylor raised over $5000 in support of the American Cancer Society. THANK YOU to everyone who helped make that happen. Thank you to everyone who walked on the team, those who traveled to be a part of it. It seemed like a whirlwind, but it really meant a lot to see the support for Team Princess Taylor and the American Cancer Society overall. We had some hard core folks who stayed out there all night, and I think Luke (Taylor's cousin) gets the award for 'Most Energy' of any team member out there! He never stopped going all night (whether it was walking the track, playing football, taking a pie in the face, doing the morning Zumba routine....it was pretty impressive!) Grandpa is a close tie with his commitment of walking 5 hours straight!

Taylor was excited about the event- although a little over-whelmed as well. She withdraws a little bit with all of the attention, so we didn't force her to 'do' anything she didn't want to. She opted not to do the survivor lap or the survivor picture- and that's okay. If it's too much for her, we don't want to push her. We had to cut her participation a little short due to Shands calling to let us know her counts were running low (we had taken her to KidsKorner to get her counts checked at noon the day of the Relay). We were literally pulling in to the Relay parking lot when Rob got the phone call that her counts were down in the 300 range. Needless to say, it is concerning, as she is neutropenic (meaning she is extremely susceptible to infection at the moment) and resulted in us going back to 'quarantine' mode for a while. Her doctors are holding her daily chemo at the moment, and she'll stay out of school this week until we have her counts checked and see if they rebound. The trip to Dancing with the Stars may be on hold (pending her counts coming back up), but we will see how her counts are this week. The good news is that she is eating and drinking and has a lot of energy- so there are things to be thankful for, and we just pray that she gets past this bump in the road, avoids a hospital stay, and keeps on progressing through the remaining 11 months of treatment.

Thank you to everyone who has called and checked in on us. We'll keep you posted on her progress this week. I am happy that she will be seeing her doctors at Shands next week for her monthly checkup.

Love, Rob, Kim, Taylor, and Alex

April 18, 2008

Taylor's strength continues to amaze us (and Germy is doing his job!!!) We took her to get her counts checked on Wednesday and they had skyrocketed up to over 900. While she has been in good spirits all week, her counts had said something different at the end of last week when they were down around 300....so we were thankful to see her rebound so quickly. We kept her out of school the remainder of the week to let her strength continue to build (and to stay away from any yucky germs).... Now that her counts are up, her doctors have resumed her daily chemo at half the dose. When they see her next week at Shands and assess her counts at that point, they will decide on what dosage to proceed with.

So with that said- her trip to California is still on for this weekend. She came home and started packing once we got back from KidsKorner (on Wednesday) and got the okay from her doctors about going!

We'll take lots of pictures and keep everyone posted on her

progress this week, including her trip to Shands.

Update from California: Taylor, Grandma, and Mommy made it out here safely. It was a long day traveling, but Taylor's excitement kept her going strong. Rob stayed home with Alex, as we felt this trip would still be tough on her (being so young), but my heart is breaking not having them both out here with us, especially since today was Rob's birthday. We miss them both very much!!! We'll take lots of pictures, and Taylor is looking forward to attending a dress rehearsal for Dancing with the Stars on Monday. Love to all, and thank you again for all of your prayers...Love, Rob, Kim, Taylor, and Alex

April 29, 2008

Sorry for the delay in updating, but it has been a busy, busy week! Let me start by saying that the trip to Hollywood was wonderful. I can't say enough about the wonderful folks at Dancing with the Stars, and the invitation for Taylor to attend the dress rehearsal last Monday. It was different from her last visit, as this was a dress rehearsal the day of the show (with the dancers in their full dress for the show and the announcers practicing their lines), so it was really neat to see the show from that perspective too.

Thank you very much to Grandma who made the trip out there with us. We packed a lot into a few days- Disneyland, American Girl Cafe and doing a self-guided tour of the stars' homes (Grandma found a good map at the store :) We also made a stop at a fire station in Bel Air where the firefighters were kind enough to give us a shirt for Daddy (so he has one from LA now too). Taylor had a good time visiting the fire station, and chatting with the firefighters there...The trip was a good time, and Taylor was a good traveler- I'm really happy we were able to do this.

Once we got back in town, it continued to be a busy week. Taylor and Rob headed down to Shands for her monthly visit. Her counts were above 700, but her doctors are holding her at a half dose of her daily chemo right now (as a full dose would probably cause the counts to drop again). On Friday, she started her 5 day steroid stint, and it has been a rough one. Things will go well for a while, and then the littlest thing will set her off. It's hard to explain to someone who hasn't gone through this- but it's almost as if she 'hangs on' to something and just can't let it go- no matter how small. For example, she went into a 1 hour rage last night over a blanket, and the fact that she wanted her Daddy to go get it (and not Mommy). Typically, you would tell a child to get over it and stop whining. We can't give into it just because she's on steroids, so you tell her the same thing, but instead of getting over it in 5 minutes, it takes an hour or so- and then she just ends up crying herself to sleep. Rob and I remind ourselves that we are happy she is still here with us- to yell and scream and fight- it is just a rough week each month....but we'll get through it. Today is Tuesday and the last day of her steroid stint, so we are happy.

We will keep everyone posted on her progress, and the countdown continues- a little over 10 months to go of treatment!

Love to all...love, Rob, Kim, Taylor, and Alex

May 13, 2008

Taylor's counts rebounded tremendously (an ANC over 2100 as of last Thursday), and her doctors have increased her daily chemo dose to 75%. Her other blood count levels were at acceptable levels too, so we continue to be thankful. We'll head to Gainesville next week for her monthly checkup at which time they'll decide whether to increase the chemo dosage even more (as they try to get her back to 100%). She has a ton of energy which Rob and I continue to be thankful for....he and I were even chatting the other day that sometimes you'd never know she was even going through all of this (with the exception of steroids!!!)

There are mini-milestones throughout this whole process,

and as of our visit this month, we will be at 10 months until her end of treatment date. So, to find little things to keep us motivated, I remind myself that after this month, we will be in the 'single digits' of the countdown!

Speaking of milestones, Miss Taylor attended her Kindergarten orientation a couple of weeks ago and is getting ready for her Pre-K graduation. While these would have been milestones regardless, it just means so much more right now. 16 months ago when she was first in the hospital- you find yourself wondering if she'll ever know a normal life again, and now it is just so reassuring to see her doing so many 'normal' things!

We spent Mother's Day weekend in Port Saint Lucie to visit Gammy (Rob's mom). Gammy was in the hospital, but thankfully was able to come home Saturday evening (in time for Mother's Day). We continue to pray that her health improves and are trying to plan our next visit down so that the girls can spend more time with Gammy outside of the hospital. Aunt Kathy and I took the girls and Cousin Luke to a water fountain park near Port Saint Lucie, and they had a blast this weekend. It was a good break from the hospital for the kids, and it gave Rob some one on one time with his Mom. The kids loved running through the fountain and playing on the beach. We came home to Tallahassee on Sunday and had a chance to have dinner with Grandma and Grandpa. It was a nice weekend with family...

Hope all of the moms had a wonderful Mother's Day, and we will keep you posted on Taylor's progress this week. Love to all....

Love, Rob, Kim, Taylor, and Alex

May 25, 2008

Taylor had her big recital yesterday, and it was just wonderful. It was wonderful for so many reasons- to see her be so brave and do her recital dance in front of a full auditorium, and the fact that her hair was long enough to pull back so that she looked like all of the other little girls in class (It is AMAZING what you can do with enough hair gel and bobby pins). I would be lying if I said that Rob and I hadn't been worried all week about how the recital would go (as she is on her steroid stint right now)- but everything went just fine! She had her dress rehearsal on Friday afternoon- after which she told us that she really wants to do tap and ballet class now....somehow getting on the stage to practice made her love dancing even more. And she did just great at the show on Saturday- It was really adorable.

Taylor also had her visit to Shands this past Thursday, and her counts were over 2800. Her other blood counts were at acceptable levels as well, so her doctors have resumed her daily chemo to 100%. In fact, they bumped up her 6-MP by another half pill once per week. Visits to clinic have been pretty tough lately- I say all of that from afar, as Rob has been the one taking the brunt of that the past few months. Taylor fights going to clinic, and fights getting her buddy accessed while she is there. It's so different from a year ago. She kicks, screams, cries, fights....we think she is just over it all. That is also what the doctors and nurses told Rob. They said "She's a year older now- she is much more aware of everything going on...she's tired of this." I can't really blame her...27 months of treatment would be tough on anyone, but especially a kid...Before Taylor had cancer, I will admit that I was ignorant to the various types of treatment. I just assumed that with cancer- you went for chemo for a few months and then back for some checkups, but I had no idea of the constant medicine regimen and steroids and stress. I was definitely sheltered from all of that, but understandably have a new appreciation for it all now.

While we can't read her mind, you do see her getting to a frustration point with all of this. When she got home on Thursday from clinic, we had dinner, and she just all of a sudden says "Mommy, I wish I never got cancer." It stopped us dead in conversation as we wanted to be careful about what we said next. I just looked at her and said "I can understand that Taylor." Rob and I tried to talk to her about it a little more and see if she would open up a bit- but she wouldn't. She seems to open up in other ways though. I was talking to one of the child life specialists here in town, and she asked me if Taylor does any role playing. I chuckled a little and explained to her that Taylor has remodeled her bedroom closet into a 'baby hospital.' She has cribs and babies and toys...and decorations on the wall...and all of her babies have procedures and have to take 'spicy, yucky medicine.' She told us it was healthy for Taylor to do that. I will admit that at first I wasn't sure if I should encourage it, so it was nice to have that validation.

Rob also had a chance to catch up with one of the teenagers at clinic this week. It was very enlightening actually- as he was able to explain to Rob the things that Taylor can't explain to us. Rob asked him about being on steroids, and he explained to Rob how much of a struggle it is. He explained to Rob that he was awake at one point for almost a week straight. (That put it into better perspective when we can't get Taylor to sleep until 11 or 12 at night- even with Benadryl). He also talked about uncontrollable food cravings- eating an entire box of Corn Flakes at a sitting- it's like he was interpreting a lot of things for us- things that Taylor hasn't been able to explain to us.

All of that said, we are in the single digits now...only 9 months and 27 days or so until March 22, 2009 (her end of treatment date). So, while these frustrations come up- we also remember how far we've come, and the amazing progress that Taylor continues to make. We will keep you posted on her progress this week, including her big milestone of Pre-K graduation!!!

Love to all....Love, Rob, Kim, Taylor and Alex

May 31, 2008

Last night was Taylor's big VPK graduation (graduation from pre-school). While she will still be at Scottsdale for the summer session, the 'official' VPK year wrapped up with graduation yesterday. The graduation was just wonderful, and the kids were just beaming with pride. They really were- all of them were so happy on stage, and they all did such a good job singing their songs and reciting their various lines. They all looked so comfortable up there in front of the crowd....it was really such a testament to the teachers and how much love they have for the kids...I can't say enough about how amazing Scottsdale and their staff are. I am so happy that is where Taylor and Alex have both spent their pre-school years.

I think I was on the verge of tears the entire evening- There was a sweet video that the teachers put together (with the kids' baby pictures and current pictures), and the kids read their journal entries about "What they are looking forward to about Kindergarten." There was lots of singing...and of course they received diplomas too! I was just so proud of Taylor and of course I couldn't help but just breathe deeply and think of yet another milestone she is hitting in her young life. It was also a bittersweet time because all of her little friends will be splitting up now and going to different schools, but I explained to Taylor that she will make new friends too when she gets to Kindergarten.

Rob and I are excited to say that Taylor wrapped up her steroid stint this week. All in all, this was probably the best steroid stint since last September. There were outbursts, but overall it was very manageable. Her appetite was huge, but we've come to expect that now. I actually held off on going food shopping to replace some of the things she was eating so much of (just so that we could honestly say "Taylor- there are no more cheese sticks.") Her appetite seems to be back to normal now, and within the next couple of days she should be able to get to bed a little easier at night too. It just seems to take a few days for all of the steroid effects to subside.

And a big thank you to the nice firefighter who covered a couple of hours for Rob so that he could attend Taylor's graduation last night before going on shift....Taylor was thrilled that he was able to come. I told her that he would not miss it for the world...

We'll continue to keep you posted on her progress and the march to the end of treatment date (March 2009!!!)

Love to all....Love, Rob, Kim, Taylor, and Alex

June 12, 2008

Just a quick update to say Hello and let everyone know that Taylor has had a great week. We took some time to head down to Orlando last week, and we also had a chance to spend some time in Port Saint Lucie.

It was a nice family trip, and we all got a little spoiled getting to spend so much time together! We posted some pictures- the girls had a blast!

Taylor has her 2 day trip to Gainesville next week, and she is getting anxious about it. It's crazy- because we don't even bring it up, but she is just constantly thinking about it. We are trying to stay positive about it when she brings it up, and are trying to distract her by talking about going to see a movie or something. It's not like there is a choice, so we will just do our best to help her get through it. Each trip brings her one month closer to being done with treatment though!!! So, we just continue to march forward. We'll keep everyone posted on her trip, and thank you again for all of your prayers and kind words on the website....

Love to all...

Love, Rob, Kim, Taylor, and Alex

June 20, 2008

It has not been an easy morning- it's been a hard couple of days actually, but this morning was really hard.

As I've mentioned recently, Taylor is very anxious about

clinic trips, but she is especially anxious about any over-night stays where a procedure (such as her lumbar puncture) is involved. Rob and I talked about various ways to try and ease the anxiety for this month's overnight trip, including making 2 day trips (instead of staying overnight). While it may have helped some, she was still pretty anxious.

Grandma and I took Taylor to clinic yesterday, and we eventually got her inside the building without too much trouble (only a few minutes of her threatening to lock herself in the car and never come out). We finally talked her into just taking baby steps (Let's get out of the car....okay, now let's walk into the building, etc.) The child life specialist (Miss Jenna) also met us and spent a lot of time with Taylor trying to talk through what is making her so nervous and trying various distraction techniques to get her mind off of everything. The most successful thing was a 'jewelry making session' where Jenna helped Taylor make a beautiful beaded necklace (with glow in the dark beads too!) Jenna explained the rules....that while Taylor and her were making the necklace-they couldn't talk about the procedure on Friday. It really worked- it calmed her down enough to get through the remaining 3 hours we were at clinic, and we didn't touch on the subject again until we wrapped up and checked out. I also spoke to her doctor about her anxiety, and he prescribed a sedative to give her this morning before she and Rob hit the road for Gainesville (at 5:30 a.m.). Her ANC was at 730, and her other counts were at acceptable levels. The 730 seemed a little low, but her steroids should help to boost her a little bit this weekend. After clinic, we went to the Butterfly Rainforest for a visit, and it seemed to keep Taylor's mind off the fact that her buddy was still accessed and that she had to head back to Gainesville on Friday- but that was only short lived....she couldn't get it off her mind when we got home last night.

So, back to this morning. We waited until the last possible

minute to get her out of bed, as we knew it would be miserable....and it was. As we picked her up, she started mumbling in a sleepy voice "I won't go to Gainesville- I'm not going, just let me sleep in my bed." The crying and screaming just elevated as we carried her to the car (sedative in hand, but let me tell you- not so easy to give a screaming 4 year old a pill to swallow in the midst of all of this). Finally, we got her to take it (and hopefully the neighbors eventually got back to sleep), but she was clinging to me saying "I don't want to go. Don't leave me Mommy, come with me, please!" It broke my heart to get out of the van and watch them drive away, but I had to.

How do you explain to your daughter that you want to come but that other life is still going on around you? Work, getting Alex to school, etc.- I hope that the medicine truly works and that Rob doesn't have 2 hours of screaming ahead of him during the drive, but it wasn't looking that way.

The doctors don't have a specific explanation as to why she is so anxious now (when the majority of time over the past 18 months was not this painful)- although they just reiterated that she is a year older, and much more cognizant of everything going on. I reminded Rob yesterday that 9 months from Sunday will be the end of treatment date. I told him- we can do this- it's not even as long as a pregnancy, and we've gone through 2 of those! (as every Mom knows that a pregnancy is REALLY 10 months....40 weeks is 10 months you know....)

All of that said- we can see the light at the end of the tunnel, and we know that Taylor has come so far on this journey. I told her last night that I never want her to forget how brave she is and how proud of her we are.

Please keep her in your prayers this morning. Her lumbar puncture (spinal chemo) procedure is at 8:50. Following that, and time (and mood) permitting, she and Rob may head to the Butterfly Rainforest and then back to Tallahassee. We're bracing for a steroid weekend, but it gets us one stint closer to March....

Love to all, and I'll keep you posted on her progress.

Love, Rob, Kim, Taylor and Alex

June 24, 2008

Thank you to everyone for your kind words of support and prayers. I wanted to update sooner, but it has been pretty busy. To pick up where I left off last week, Rob and Taylor made it to Gainesville- she screamed for a while (I guess until the sedative kicked in), and

then slept for the remainder of the trip. In the midst of everything going on Friday morning, we had forgotten to put a pair of shoes in the car for her. Ironically though, when she and Rob got to Gainesville and to the surgery center- she giggled about having no shoes while Rob carried her inside. It was good to hear she was giggling.

Rob said she did okay overall- they gave her some extra medicine to calm her down, and then did her procedure. The procedure doesn't take long, but you can imagine that with all of her 'calming down' medicine-it just took a while to wake up! Even so, Rob and Taylor made it home to Tallahassee by early afternoon and in time for lunch at Boston Market (one of her favorite places to eat).

She has been on her steroids, and we are thankful that the side effects have been minimal (comparatively to other months). There are still the food cravings and outbursts, but they seem to be slightly better in check than in months past. Today is Tuesday, and the last day of steroids for the month, so we are very happy!

I had the chance to attend the Relay for Life wrap-up dinner last night, and was so proud that Team Princess Taylor was a part of the Relay this year. Our little event raised $87,000 over 41 teams! It was inspiring and of course makes you look ahead to next year and how to do it all over again! I was very flattered and humbled that Team Princess Taylor also received 3 awards (including one for our Sweet Shop- the chocolate awareness ribbons that Miss Kathryn made for the team). Thank you again to everyone for their participation with Team Princess Taylor. It does make a difference!

We will keep everyone posted on her progress. The countdown to the end of her chemotherapy is definitely on now....as of last Sunday, there are 9 months to go- meaning we are at 8 months and some days now :)

Take care, and have a good week!

Love, Rob, Kim, Taylor, and Alex

July 10, 2008

It has been a great couple of weeks. I hope everyone had a wonderful 4th of July- it is truly one of Taylor's favorite holidays. She and Alex were planning their outfits for a week! They also made a yummy 'American flag' cake with lots of strawberries and blueberries. In addition to a busy 4th, we also had Taylor's 5th birthday party last Saturday. Her birthday is actually on the 12th, but the pool was available last weekend....so she got to be 5 a whole week early (at least that is what she is telling me).

The pool party was great, and the weather was perfect. She wanted to have a princess party, and helped pick out all of the decorations and desserts. She and her daddy made all of the goody bags together too. She asked the lady at the bakery for frosting with sprinkles and princess rings...everything was great. She has also started swim lessons this week- so there has been a lot going on!

Taylor has been doing well overall, and will make her trip to Gainesville for her checkup next week. She hasn't brought it up in the past couple of days, and we will try not to bring it up until the absolute last minute. No need for her to be anxious....

We will keep everyone posted, and appreciate all of your postings and kind words. We are getting close to the 8 month mark- her end of chemo gets closer each day!!!

Love to all, and we'll keep you posted on her progress this week. Love, Rob, Kim, Taylor, and Alex

July 12, 2008

Taylor had a great birthday....as Rob says, it feels like she's had a 'birthday week....'- between her birthday last weekend, cupcakes at school this week, and then her actual birthday today- but that's just fine with me.

We had a really busy and fun day today, starting off with a hair appointment with Alex and Taylor's friend Riley. It's pretty cute to see 3 little girls at the hair salon together- getting all dolled up. Following their appointment, the girls headed to their friend Jenna's birthday party, and then we spent the afternoon swimming. We had told Taylor that we would focus on doing a birthday dinner when her Daddy got home from the fire station tonight. We told her she could pick to go out to dinner wherever she wanted (or we could make a favorite dinner at home). She picked Boston Market. I asked her if she was sure, and she was, so Boston Market it was....sometimes you have to appreciate simplicity! After dinner, she opened up her presents from Rob, Alex, and I. She has been asking for a fish for about 2 months now, so she was happy to open up a fish tank and all of the accessories....now all she is missing is the fish. Her daddy is going to take her to the pet store tomorrow.

As I read books to her tonight, she was pretty tired- but she hung on for 3 books before falling asleep. She looked like a little angel sleeping. I took a minute just to watch her and give thanks for another birthday. I gave her a kiss and said a quick prayer to thank God for where she is today. She is a strong, strong little girl.

A funny note about the hair salon....Taylor is on a kick about growing out her bangs. There have been days recently where she doesn't want to pull her bangs back, and they are hanging in her eyes...so I was hoping she would agree to just trim her bangs up a little bit today at the salon. Then I reminded myself- "It's just hair." That is what I told myself a year ago when she was completely bald, so I shouldn't think any differently now! If she wants to grow it down to her toes, who cares?

Thank you to everyone for your birthday wishes for Taylor. We will keep you posted on her visit to Shands this week. Love to all....Love, Rob, Kim, Taylor, and Alex

July 22, 2008

Happy Tuesday! (And the last day of this month's steroid stint!) I continue to be amazed at Taylor's ability to push through these tough stints. Not to say this weekend wasn't without a couple of tantrums / outbursts and a noticeable appetite increase, but we've all made it through in one piece!

Overall, she continues to be full of energy, and had a great trip to Gainesville with her Daddy last Thursday to get her IV chemo (Vincristine), lab work, and her monthly checkup. Her ANC was over 1400, so her daily chemo is staying at its current 100% level. Her platelets, white blood cells, hematocrit, and hemoglobin all looked within acceptable levels too, so she'll just keep on marching through this! Many thanks to her doctors who are adjusting next month's IV chemo / steroid stint to NOT coincide with the first day of Kindergarten. Instead, they are pushing back her doses until the following week. Rob and I were very appreciative, as the first day of Kindergarten may cause its own set of anxiety (and the steroids increase her anxiety), so this will make it a little easier on little Miss Taylor as she moves on to big kid school...

I love the picture of Aunt Debbie and the girls on the boat- we've spent some time over the past couple of weekends taking the kids to play at the beach on Dog Island (a fun little place right off the coast for those not familiar with North Florida :), and it has just been some really good family time. The kids love it and have a great time finding shells, making sand castles, and just splashing. Alex woke up yesterday morning and asked 'Can we go to Dog Island again today Mommy?' I told her we'll have to wait for the weekend, but was glad to see that she has such a good time. I love spending time with the kids outside, on the boat- just keeping them active and busy....especially on a steroid weekend when it keeps Taylor distracted from eating non-stop. Plus, we're all getting great tans. Taylor is also practicing all of her new moves from swim lessons. She finished up a 2 week swim lesson session last week....and although there were a couple nights that she was kicking and screaming about going, we didn't back down, and I'm so glad we didn't. I can't say enough about the folks she went to (Bob Ruth Aquatics). She is actually swimming (something she couldn't do 2 weeks ago). I'm not saying she's doing laps in the pool yet, but what an amazing difference! Somewhere on his website, I read that swimming is 75% about confidence. If 2 weeks of lessons have given her more confidence- then even better. She is very proud of herself, and even got a ribbon on her last night of lessons (which she has hung on her wall). Rob and I told her that we are proud that she finished what she started.

We will keep you posted on her progress and the days leading up to Kindergarten!!! My mom gave the girls and I a great gift the other night. It was a picture of me when I started Kindergarten (just a few years ago...). She gave the girls a frame with 2 placeholders for pictures. On the left side, she put the picture of me on the first day of Kindergarten, and she left a place on the right for their picture when they start Kindergarten. The ironic thing about the picture is that Taylor's hair is actually slightly longer than mine was when I started Kindergarten (about 6-7 months before Kindergarten, Aunt Debbie and I had played 'hairdresser', and mom had no choice but to give us both buzz cuts....so by the time Kindergarten started, it was just getting to a decent length). It's funny how God gives you those moments. Taylor and I looked at the picture together, and I told her- "You and Mommy sure do look a lot alike. We have similar hairstyles." and she said "We sure do!"

Thank you for your continued prayers. As of today, Taylor is within the 8 month timeframe for the end of chemo. It's hard to say there is ever an end to any of this, as there will always be the ongoing appointments and testing to make sure the cancer stays away- but we will take the milestones as they come, and will give thanks for each of them!

Love to all....

Love, Rob, Kim, Taylor, and Alex

August 10, 2008

Only 1 week until Taylor starts Kindergarten! This week will be a big week- filled with orientations, meeting her Kindergarten teacher, goodbyes to her friends at Scottsdale....lots of things! She is getting a little nervous, but Rob and I remind her that when she started at Scottsdale, she only knew a couple of people, and she made lots of new friends. I also remind her that it is normal to feel a little nervous, and that Mommy did too when she started Kindergarten. We're keeping an eye on her counts, and her labs looked good on Wednesday at Kids Korner- her ANC was around 1500, and her platelets, hematocrit and hemoglobin were at good levels too. We're holding off on going to Gainesville this week for Vincristine (her IV chemo) and will be going next week instead. This helps to keep her off of steroids for the first week of school, and just moves her IV chemo by 1 week. Most likely, we will resume her normal schedule, and go back to Gainesville 3 weeks later (instead of the normal 4 weeks), but that will keep her on track for her end of treatment date.

As I looked through some photos tonight, I realized that Miss Taylor has kept pretty busy this summer- complete with family vacation time, spending time with friends, lots of water days at school, and pool parties. I took this past week off of work, and Rob and I did a long weekend vacation dur-

225

ing the first part of the week, and then the girls and I took some time later this week to do a 'girls' trip to Alabama to see our friends Miss Kathryn, Mr. Bart, Kaitlyn and Tori. The girls had a blast playing on the swing set and swimming with Kaitlyn and Tori- and were excited to see some sights in Alabama too. I managed to teach them a few lines of 'Sweet Home Alabama' along the way too....Taylor also understands the rivalry now between Auburn and Alabama (and that it is similar to how the Gators feel about the Seminoles). Mommy did make a boo-boo with our Alabama trip- I forgot to double check Taylor's medicine prior to leaving, so thank god for Walgreens....as we were running low on Methotrexate (one of her chemo meds that she takes once per week). We managed to find a Walgreens in Albertville, Alabama who had it in stock though, so we didn't miss a beat.

Miss Kathryn was kind enough to make Grandma a yummy birthday cake, and it made it back to Tallahassee in one piece! We celebrated Grandma's birthday tonight with a cookout and birthday cake, and then Taylor settled in with Grandpa to watch the Olympics. She is absolutely in love with watching the women's gymnastics (as I'm sure most little girls are!) She fought to stay awake to finish watching Team USA, but fell asleep....thankfully there will be a lot more to watch!

She continues to amaze us each day, and I try to always remember to be thankful for the little things (as well as the big things). Starting Kindergarten is a huge thing to be thankful for- but then there are also times like today when I was watching her run and play outside, and I remember to be thankful for her muscles continuing to stay strong. We will keep everyone posted on her progress this week, the first day of school, and her trip to Gainesville next week too. Thank you for your continued prayers- I truly believe that those prayers are what help these little miracles continue to happen for Taylor.

Love to all....

Love, Rob, Kim, Taylor, and Alex

August 18, 2008

So today was the big first day of Kindergarten, and Miss Taylor loved it! She has a wonderful teacher, and while she had a couple bouts of nerves this morning, she handled it well. She paused a bit before going into class, but after a little encouragement, she walked into the classroom and did just fine. She saw her friend Christopher, and that made her smile. After a couple of quick hugs and kisses (and showing Alex and Daddy the class iguana....), we left....and she didn't look back. It was amazing. After leaving elementary school, we dropped Alex off at her new class at school, and she was a champ too...a little clingy, but no tears- and we were off to our boo-hoo breakfast.

We couldn't wait to hear about the kids' days at school- and Taylor was upset that Rob picked her up so 'early' from aftercare...she told him "Daddy, we were headed to the playground!" He and I took that as a good sign that she liked school. After reading books tonight (including her first library book that she already got to check out!), I asked Taylor what her favorite thing was about Kindergarten today, and she told me "Everything." I was so happy....

It was a busy week leading up to Kindergarten, including some scares with Taylor's blood sugar, but all appears to be okay at the moment. She was having some frequent bouts of low blood sugar last week, and Shands had us take her for various labs, including something called a Hemoglobin A1C test to check for treatment-induced Diabetes (I'm pretty sure that's how you spell the name of the test!) Basically, the test provides a 3 month view of her blood sugars, and gives the mean value of the blood sugar for those 3 months. This provides a bigger picture perspective as opposed to just a finger stick to show a point in time test of her levels. In short- her levels were fine, and some of the nausea may be continuing side effects from the chemo. We'll continue to keep an eye on it, and raise any concerns to her doctors- which we will see this week during her check- up visit.

All in all though, things continue to progress, and we are getting closer to March, 2009 (her end of treatment date). She will get her IV chemo this week (the Vincristine) and have her steroid stint, but it was nice for her to not have the emotional stress of the steroids this week as she started school. We'll manage the steroid stint as it comes this week, and are just thankful that her doctors were able to delay it for the first day of school.

We'll keep you posted on her checkup this week, and thank you again for your prayers.

Love, Rob, Kim, Taylor, and Alex

August 23, 2008

Taylor and Alex had a great first week of school. Alex is adjusting to life at Scottsdale without Taylor, although she was a little sad the first couple of days, and Taylor came home every day this week excited about her day at Kindergarten. The kids had Friday off from school due to Tropical Storm Fay (and possibly this coming Monday, but hopefully all will be okay by then).

Since Tropical Storm Fay has taken her time coming across the state of Florida, Rob and Taylor hit some of the bad weather on the way to and from Gainesville as well on Thursday. Taylor had a good clinic visit- with her ANC over 1300, and hemoglobin, hematocrit, and platelet counts all at acceptable levels too. Rob and I initially thought that because her ANC has been at a high level, the doctors may increase her chemo dosage, but they said they only do that if it stays at a high level for an extended period of time. So, that was good to hear. They did increase her antibiotic dosage (for the Septra she takes on the weekends), but that was due to the fact that she is a growing girl and the dosage factors in weight as well. Rob said that Taylor was not anxious at clinic or about having her 'buddy' accessed, but that she was clear that "this is only a 1 day trip, right Daddy??? I'm not staying overnight!!!" Thankfully, he was able to tell her that it was only a 1 day trip. Next month, that's a different story because she'll have to stay overnight for her lumbar puncture (spinal chemo) procedure on Friday morning. We'll take one day at a time though, and deal with that as it gets closer.

I'd ask that everyone say an extra prayer for Rob and his family. Rob's mom has been in and out of the hospital a good bit this year, and has been back in this past week. She is a strong lady (I can tell where Rob gets it from :) He does an amazing job balancing everything going on in our own household as well as making trips to be with his Mom, but I know it's tough. We pray that Gammy will be well enough to come home, and that the kids will be able to spend some time with her soon.

We'll keep everyone posted on Taylor's progress, and her continued excitement about school! As of yesterday, she is 7 months away from the end of treatment....which means today she is 6 months and 30 days away...with each day, the countdown gets better and better. Love to all, and thank you for your prayers and postings.

Love, Rob, Kim, Taylor, and Alex

September 2, 2008

Things continue to progress here in the Koegel household! Another week of school is complete, and we are already on to week 3 of Kindergarten! With week 3 comes Taylor's first taste of homework, and it is too cute- she is so excited about it! She has 'homework' assignments Monday through Thursday and then turns her folder into her teacher on Friday. Tonight's assignment was practicing writing her name 3 times and counting to 20. We are also working on sight words- it is wonderful to see her so excited about learning words and wanting to read! She truly is loving school, and we count our blessings that everything feels so 'normal' sometimes.

We will head to Gainesville next week for a 2 day visit- the first day will be her clinic visit with IV chemo (the Vincristine) and her checkup with her doctors. Day 2 will be her early morning lumbar puncture (the spinal chemo). Rob and I don't know what to expect next week. She is so anxious recently about clinic visits, especially anything with an overnight stay. We'll just take it day by day though and try to manage her anxiety as best we can. The amazing thing is that after next week's lumbar puncture, she will only have 2 more left during treatment! That is amazing! I remember early on during treatment when she had a lumbar puncture at least once per week. It is frightening to think just how aggressive this cancer can be. For those that may have not been following the site early on- lumbar punctures are the method by which the doctors administer chemotherapy via the spine. During the procedure, they also retain a bit of spinal fluid to make sure it is 'clear' (meaning that the cancer has not traveled to Taylor's brain).

Aside from some red bumps on her face (caused as a side effect from her Methotrexate), Taylor continues to march through treatment. She notices the bumps on her face, but seems to ignore them for the most part. I hate that she has to endure any additional side effects, but it is what it is. Taylor's doctors are also having us give her Zofran each night before bed to help with the nausea in the morning- this has seemed to help tremendously. We are also quick to get her something to eat and drink first thing when she wakes up. This has seemed to help keep her nausea away, so we are happy.

Alex and Taylor both start dance class tomorrow, so they are very excited....especially Miss Alex as this is her first time taking a class. I took the girls this evening to get their ballet and tap shoes as well as a new leotard each- it was precious watching them try on everything. I just try to soak it all in and treasure these times- I'm sure they will fly by!

We will keep everyone posted on Taylor's continued progress and her trip to Gainesville next week (and the ongoing homework assignments too!) Love to all....

Love, Rob, Kim, Taylor, and Alex

September 10, 2008

Rob and Taylor head to Gainesville tomorrow. We sat down and talked to Taylor about it tonight, and while it took a little bit for her to come around- her suitcase is finally packed, and she helped do it.

She doesn't want to go- and it took some discussion about a special "date night with Daddy," and possibly a trip to Build a Bear while they are in Gainesville as a special treat- but we prefer to do these 'special treats' all day long as opposed to having to sedate her again to go. Rob tried to explain to her tonight that he wishes we had a choice in the matter, but we don't- he explained that it is important for her to go and get the medicine she needs. Somehow, she must have been able to process enough to help start packing the suitcase- and even picked out her "date night" dress for tomorrow night. We'll just take baby steps and get her to clinic tomorrow for her IV chemo and her checkup, and then we'll go from there. Friday morning will be the tough part, as she gets anxious about the lumbar puncture (the spinal tap procedure where she is asleep and they give her the chemo in her spine); but when she gets past Friday, there are only 2 more of these left during her treatment.

She and Alex are having fun at dance class, and they were thrilled that Daddy came straight from his shift to see them tonight. Taylor continues to enjoy Kindergarten, and is excited about all of the new things she is learning....We filled this past weekend with lots of FSU football festivities, including the Downtown Getdown on Friday night and an attempted trip to the first football game on Saturday. The game was on a 2 hour rain / lightning delay, so we didn't stay, but thankfully we avoided the rain altogether. In general, I like to avoid getting soaked at games- but it takes on a whole new meaning when you are scared of your child catching a cold that could turn into something much worse....so Rob and I were okay with a quick exit from the game and staying dry!

The important thing to us is that we try to keep everything as normal as we can for her though- school, dance, heading to football games, playing with her friends- it's all part of her leading a normal life....and we are just hopeful that in a little more than 6 months, she can be done with most of this. The worry will never stop. We know that. In fact, I wish I could explain just how much we know that- how hard it is to go to clinic and see the suffering going on with these young, innocent children- of all ages, different cancers, cases of relapse, hoping for a match of a bone marrow transplant-different stories, worried parents- all hoping for some magic drug to make it go away. But even when the chemotherapy is done, there isn't a statistic that makes it 100% better. Sure, the odds are better for certain types of cancer vs. others, but nothing is 100%, and you truly do have to turn everything over to God to get any sort of peace about the whole thing and that there is a reason for all of it. I think that's why we like to hear the success stories out there- the 30 year old who had Leukemia when they were a child and are now living a 'normal' life all these years later. It's not that we want to have blinders on and not hear the bad news- but we already have enough on our plate to get through each day without being reminded of the uncertainties ahead, the children dying way before their time. Believe me, we know it's out there- we know things can change on a dime- we see it every day- but sometimes it takes everything you have to put on a good face and put those worries out of your mind. The alternative though is to be sad about it all the time- so putting on a good face and trying to be positive and having faith seems like the better plan to us. Rob and I will continue to do what's best for Taylor- keep a positive attitude and get through this.

We will keep everyone posted on Taylor's trip to Gainesville this week. Please keep her and Rob in your prayers as they travel and as Rob tries to calm her nerves and prepare her for her procedures over the next 2 days. Love to all, and thank you again for all of your postings and notes. Love, Rob, Kim, Taylor, and Alex

September 12, 2008

Rob and Taylor made it back from Gainesville safely today. All in all, the trip went well. Rob said that Taylor had minimal anxiety about things- she did fine at clinic, had a great 'date night with Daddy,' and slept well at the hotel last night too. Mommy must have a mental block with sending the right shoes in her suitcase though. Rob and I were laughing on the phone last night- because Taylor put on her beautiful 'date night ' dress that she had packed....but had to wear her sneakers 'cause we had forgotten her dress shoes! This is the second time we've had a 'shoe incident' when she's headed to Gainesville, but it's good for a little laugh I guess :)

Taylor was a little hesitant about heading to the surgery center this morning for her lumbar puncture, but didn't resist too much. The procedure went fine, and they were back on the road by mid-morning to head home. Unfortunately, Taylor did have some side effects from the procedure on the way home (vomiting and upset tummy)- so the trip home took a bit longer than expected- but she progressively felt better throughout the day. By the time I got home from work, she was playing with her friends and riding her bike. Kids are amazing! Any parent with young kids knows that a cold may make a kid feel bad- but it doesn't seem to slow them down in terms of playing hard! That is all I could think about as I watched Taylor and Alex riding their bikes up and down the street tonight- what a blessing.

Her counts at clinic looked great- her ANC was over 1200, and her hematocrit, hemoglobin, and platelets were all within normal limits- that was really amazing to see. The doctors did need to bump up her steroid dosage slightly due to continuing to grow bigger and stronger! She looks so healthy though- when she was first in the hospital in January, 2007- she was down to 25 pounds. Yesterday, she weighed 44 pounds- another blessing to see her looking so healthy! While I cringed slightly when I thought of more steroids, the dosage is appropriate for her body size, so I guess that means we shouldn't expect a difference from the previous dosage. Even if there is, everything is short term, and by Tuesday- she'll be done with this stint.

So, all is well in the Koegel household. The girls are sleeping soundly, and we are getting ready for more college football this weekend....cheerleading outfits are already laid out and ready for the game.

We'll keep everyone posted on Taylor's progress this week. Thank you for all of your kind words- I hope you all know what an amazing support network you've been for our family....and how much we appreciate your thoughts and prayers.

Love, Rob, Kim, Taylor, and Alex

September 22, 2008

Today marks the 6 month countdown until the end of Taylor's chemotherapy. It is amazing.

We have had a busy week, complete with visits to see Gammy and a trip to DisneyWorld as part of the American Cancer Society's ROCK weekend (ROCK stands for 'Reaching out to Cancer Kids'). It is a great event, and provides families with access to classes and education about childhood cancer, treatments, late effects, etc. The kids had a blast (as they were in their own activities) and had the opportunity to meet other kids and siblings that were in the same type of situation. That was really the amazing thing- it was an event focused on supporting the family- the siblings, the parents and the patient. Taylor was very proud of her picture that was on the mural that was displayed at the closing breakfast (she did a picture of her and Mommy flipping pancakes). We can't thank the American Cancer Society enough for everything this weekend.

While the event was great, I think Rob and I would also agree that it was emotionally exhausting. You are definitely consumed with the gravity of the disease and the fact that even when chemotherapy is done- there is the potential for lasting effects, learning issues- things that are out of our control but that we should watch for so that we can address. For example, the chemo that Taylor is given in her spine (the IT Methotrexate) is one of the reasons that Leukemia ALL (Pre-B) has had a higher cure rate in recent years. However, it has the potential to cause harmful side effects to the body, including her brain development. It might happen, it might not, and we may not see the effects for a few years- even if everything is okay right now. Rob was my rock and calmed me down...because I felt like I just wanted to kick a wall or something after leaving one of the sessions. I just felt like so many things were out of our control....and then I remembered that kicking the wall wouldn't really fix any of it, so I just took a deep breath and told God that I would do my best to try and conquer things as they come, and that we will continue to watch for any side effects that may come in the out years....but it does take a toll on you sometimes.

We learned something this weekend that will help us get through the steroid stints though...(Trying to find that silver lining....) In a discussion with one of the doctors about steroids, the doctor mentioned to Rob that if he had one drug to treat Leukemia with, it would be Decadron (the steroid that Taylor is currently on). He explained that the Decadron literally blows up the Leukemia cells....and that it is a drug that passes the blood / brain barrier....and some other things- but the part I kept on hearing is that it "blows up" the Leukemia cells- I will embrace this drug now!!! Every time she is having an outburst and I feel like I am going to lose my mind, I will remind myself that the drug that is doing these awful things to her is also blowing up Leukemia cells in her body to make her better. (Gotta find that silver lining).

All in all though, this weekend reminds us of how precious time is, and that we are not guaranteed tomorrow....so focus on today. Focus on being "mindful" (that was one of the sessions too)- which means that you have to live in the moment. The speaker mentioned something about how we do so many activities in a mindless fashion (e.g. driving). She reiterated that we should try to be conscious about everything we do- she mentioned something about breathing deeply at stop lights and appreciating the trees around you while you're driving- so I'll start there :) In all seriousness though, the point was well taken- we can't worry about the future- we can't control it- just try to make it through today, hug your kids and spouse tight, and pray for peace about all of this.

Rob's mom was transported to Tampa General late last week, so we were thankful to be close enough to visit on both Friday and Sunday this weekend. She is a strong lady, and we are continuing to pray for her healing as well.

We will keep everyone posted on Taylor's progress, and thank you again for keeping up with this journey...

Love, Rob, Kim, Taylor, and Alex

September 27, 2008

Last night we had a bit of a scare, and I can't say that we're quite over it just yet, but we'll get there after Monday. And before you read further, the good news is that we think everything is going to be okay and that the initial results we got were wrong.

We had Taylor's counts checked yesterday, which is a pretty standard thing. We usually get a phone call with her current ANC, hemoglobin, hematocrit, platelets, etc. Last night we got a call, and I could tell something was wrong. The nurse on the phone was explaining that the lab tech said he/she wanted a pathologist to look at the blood to confirm, but that the lab said they think they see "immature cells" in the sample. Those words may not mean anything specific to a lot of folks out there- but to a parent of a Leukemia patient, it was frightening. I asked the nurse "When you say immature, do you mean that they think they saw lymphoblasts?" And she said "yes." (which means that Leukemia cells are showing up in the sample which could signify a relapse of Taylor's cancer). My head was spinning, and I walked across the house to find Rob- the whole time coordinating with the nurse about getting the labs to Shands ASAP. Rob got on the phone to talk to the nurse as well, and within 10 minutes we were on a conference call with 3 of the pediatric hematology / oncologists from Shands.

We can't say enough about how much we appreciated how quick the doctors reacted and the attention it was given. They looked at the lab work and explained that even though Taylor's ANC was low, nothing was indicating a sign of a relapse- (remember- they are looking at everything- the hematocrit, the hemoglobin, platelets, neutrophils, etc.). The doctors got on the phone with the lab directly and clarified whether we were talking about 'atypical' cells vs. 'immature' cells (which is a HUGE difference)- and the lab tech explained that they were 'atypical.' Taylor's doctors explained that atypical cells are often present when the patient has a virus (which was completely logical because she has had a cough the past couple of days which is why we had her counts checked in the first place!) A virus can cause her counts to drop, and this is pretty common during treatment. The doctors just typically take the patient off of the daily chemo for a period of time until the counts come up again. We've been through this before with viruses during treatment to date, so it wouldn't have been a big deal to just hear that we need to hold her chemo. However, now that there was even a 'thought' about immature cells, Rob and I won't feel 100% comfortable until the doctors at Shands look at her blood under the microscope themselves.

A pathologist is looking at the blood today, but we will be taking her to clinic on Monday at Shands to get some closure on all of this.

It was a moment that I don't want to relive or have to consider in the future, but it was a glimpse into how we may actually feel if that call was to ever come. I will admit I was scared and confused, and just had to keep telling myself to not be angry- there is a reason- we can get through this- but it was definitely a little scary.

It was scary, but after the whirlwind last night, and after the kids were in bed- I think Rob and I realized that so many parents aren't given this chance. There are so many families out there that get that first call- but don't get the follow up call to say there was a mistake. We are the lucky ones.

Everything in me tells me she is okay and that she is going to be okay, and I know we will feel better after our Monday visit to Shands. I still ask that you pray for a positive outcome.

Love to all, and we will keep you posted.

Love, Rob, Kim, Taylor, and Alex

September 29, 2008

No relapse! That was the amazing news we received today at clinic! Rob and I were very relieved to hear that confirmation today, and even more relieved that Taylor was unaware that a relapse (or the gravity of it) was ever a possibility.

Taylor is still battling low counts (with an ANC of 280), but that is due to her body fighting off a nasty cold at the moment. We will keep her home from school this week (and out of public places!) as we wait for her body to rebound and we see those counts come up again. The hope is that we are able to keep her fever free, away from additional sickness, and out of the hospital as she battles these low counts.

She was not excited about going to Gainesville this morning, and specifically told us "I don't want to miss anything fun at school!" It is reassuring to know that she loves going to school each day!!! Even though she was not happy about it, she pushed through, and had a good trip though. She did great getting her buddy accessed, and was also patient while they did a chest X-ray (to rule out any pneumonia). I told her that I would check in with Mrs. Shaw (her teacher) to see if we could get her classroom assignments while she is out- and she liked that idea. Kids are too cute....

I have to let everyone know some exciting news too- Miss Taylor tied her shoes all by herself on Saturday(multiple times too!) While I was extremely proud, it was almost like a sign from God for Rob and I that everything is going to be okay. Last weekend, one of the things that came up during our sessions at ROCK weekend was that "there may be challenges with fine motor skills such as being able to tie shoes...." And then- there she was- saying "Mommy- look at me!" We needed that this past Saturday- just a reassurance that she continues to push through....What I love is that nobody told her she couldn't do it- so she's going to do everything she can! Kids are amazing...

So, all in all- you can imagine that life feels great right now in the Koegel household. We continue to appreciate every day together, and even remembered to be a little silly this weekend too (you'll have to ask Taylor about how she loves to sing 'KISS' songs while we're driving around town with the windows open). It is pretty cute to hear a 5 year old singing "I wanna rock and roll all night....." So if you thought you saw a crazy minivan of singers this weekend- it just may have been us!

Well, love to all, and thank you for all of your prayers. We will keep you posted on her progress this week and hope she is able to head back to school shortly. Love, Rob, Kim, Taylor, and Alex

October 4, 2008

Taylor had her counts checked yesterday, and they have rebounded to an ANC of 890! Her platelets, hematocrit and hemoglobin all look good too. Needless to say, we were happy- as she has continued to fight off this cold all week and we knew that the cold was taking a toll on her counts. She was not happy about having to miss school this week, so she was excited to hear she could go back on Monday....she was extra excited to hear from her teacher yesterday and to get to say 'Hi' to her on the phone. That really made her day!

We celebrated last night with a trip to Moe's for dinner (still ate outside though.....), and then a slumber party to watch 'The Wizard of Oz.' Because Taylor has not had to take her chemo this week (due to her counts being low), it has also meant that we don't have to cut off food and drinks so early in the evening (Typically, she has to eat and then wait 2 hours to take her medicine before bed). So, we even popped some popcorn last night for the movie. It's amazing how much of a treat that is for her! Daddy was on shift though, so he missed the slumber party- I'm sure he is very sad, so we'll have to do one again soon...

So, all is well for now in the Koegel household. Taylor and Alex are heading to Charlie's birthday party today and then we're probably just relaxing most of the weekend. We are hopeful that Taylor continues to feel better and are just happy that she will be able to head back to school next week.

Love to all, and we will keep you posted on her progress. Love, Rob, Kim, Taylor, and Alex

October 10, 2008

Rob and Taylor headed to Shands yesterday for Taylor's

regular monthly visit. She received her IV chemo (the Vincristine) and had her checkup with the doctors. Her counts looked fine- with an ANC over 1300. Her hematocrit, hemoglobin, and platelet counts were at acceptable levels too. They are keeping her daily chemo at 50% for now as her body continues to recover from her cold, low counts, etc. from the past couple of weeks. Her doctors will continue to monitor her counts and adjust her daily chemo back to 100% when they feel her body is ready.

Overall her visit went well. She is continuing to battle some skin effects from the medicine (the doctors tell us it is a side effect of the 6-MP and Methotrexate chemo medicines). The steroid stint this weekend should help to address some of the redness on her face, belly, etc.- but once she is off the steroids, it will come back. They also explained that once her treatment ends in March, we will probably see 2-3 months of increased skin issues due to her body trying to adjust back to a 'normal' state from the medicine, etc. It feels frustrating (you think- how much more does this kid really need to deal with?), but we'll take the skin challenges any day and I know she'll get through those just like she's gotten through so much to date. She is aware of it though (she's getting older, and I have to remember that she's aware of so much more than when all of this started). We were on our way to the fire station the other day to visit Rob, and she asked me if the firemen thought she would look funny...I asked her what she meant, and she pointed to the spot on her face. I told her that they would say what anyone would say..."What a beautiful little girl you are!" She smiled and seemed okay with that answer.

She continues to love Kindergarten, and was just thrilled to head back to school this week. She has her first field trip next week, and guess where her class is going? The fire station!!! Her daddy is chaperoning, so Taylor is extra excited about that. They are also headed to the pumpkin patch, so she is really looking forward to it.

To all of the Clemson fans out there- she watched the first part of the game last night, and was excited to see Clemson keep Wake out of the end zone (at least in the beginning). She was cheering for the defense (the only thing that kept us in the game...) She wore orange pajamas to bed- hoping that it would bring Clemson the luck they needed....unfortunately, I'll have to inform her this morning that Wake Forest was too much for the Tigers last night! She makes me laugh though- because for some reason, she has taken a liking to LSU- not sure why, but she has. She heard a commercial for LSU / Florida this weekend, and started running around the house last night cheering for LSU. "When is that game on Mommy? We'll HAVE to watch it!"

We'll keep you posted on her progress this week, and I am ready to approach this steroid stint with a whole new attitude (thanks to our ROCK weekend a few weeks back). I'm trying to think of that Decadron as blowing up everything bad in her body- and that I should be thankful that she is on it. Yeah, we'll see how this approach goes. I'll keep you posted on that too!

Love to all...Love, Rob, Kim, Taylor, and Alex

October 12, 2008

Just a quick update (and some new pictures too...) and to let everyone know that Taylor continues to amaze us.

Overall, she's done well with her steroid stint this weekend. I think she's recognizing some of her 'frustrating' feelings and chooses to spend time coloring or watching a DVD by herself- and that's fine. We all need alone time- I'm sure a 5 year old is no different! Having said that, there have been some tough times- some crying over things that may not typically warrant crying, some arguments with Alex- and definitely some challenges with insomnia. The poor kid probably only slept between 5 and 6 hours last night, and woke up around midnight absolutely starving- but it is sadly a side effect of the medicine....so I fixed her some snacks and we watched some Disney Channel until she fell asleep again. She is sleeping soundly right now though, and we are 60% of the way through her doses for this stint....we'll just take it day by day.

Thankfully, there were lots of good distractions though this weekend. Taylor and Alex spent time with Daddy down at the coast on Saturday, and then we headed to the pumpkin patch and a birthday party today. Grandma and Grandpa were working at their church pumpkin patch today, so the girls were excited to go visit them there. Taylor wasn't much for posing for pictures while we were there- but Alex posed for a few. The girls picked out 4 pumpkins (1 for each of us), and then Taylor drew faces on them when we got home today (hence the 'Koegel Pumpkin' family picture).

With any emotional outburst or hunger craving that has happened, I just think about that Decadron blowing up bad cells in her body. I will admit I had to remind myself of that tonight when the girls were going to bed and there was some crying as I was getting Taylor's medicine together and "I wasn't moving fast enough" according to Taylor, and I felt like my head was going to explode. And then I had the chance to talk to Rob, who reminds me that it is all going to pass... I said a prayer of thanks this evening though for my amazing husband and the support network we have. I can't imagine doing any of this alone. Every time I feel spent, I think of those out there doing this as single parents- or without the support structure that Rob and I have had. We are very blessed.

So- on to an exciting week at school- first field trip, school pictures....lots to do. I'm gonna head upstairs to bed and hope for a restful night. Love to all...Love, Rob, Kim, Taylor, and Alex

I know it's been awhile since the last update- but here's the latest! Taylor continues to keep busy with school, dance, and lots of 'normal' things, including traveling to Atlanta to visit with Baby Will, Charlie, Aunt Kim and Uncle Mike...and a visit up to a Clemson football game! She and Alex had a blast, and were so excited to see Kaitlyn and Tori at the game too. The girls had a teacher planning day for school the week before last, so it gave us a good chance to take a 3 day weekend and do a 'girls trip' to Atlanta and Clemson. It was a good time- complete with a trip to the American Girl Cafe in Atlanta. You can only imagine what a fun day trip that was! The girls really enjoyed it, and there was the exciting purchase of 'Kit's treehouse' which was something that we had been talking to Taylor about for a while. We had set some goals with her, and she met them, and we were very proud of her- I can chat more about that later, but I'll thank Aunt Kim for coming with us to the American Girl store. She braved the rain, bringing a newborn and a toddler (in addition to Taylor and Alex!), and helped us 'shove' the treehouse into the van in the rain. The box was pretty big, and we both ended up pretty soaked! She was a champ.

Taylor's body has continued to rebound from her low counts last month, and we had her counts checked this past Friday. Her doctors have increased her daily chemotherapy up to 75%, and then we'll be in Gainesville next week for them to see her in person. When they check her counts next week, they'll determine whether they can increase it back to 100%.

She is having a great time at school, and was excited to get to join her friend Christopher in 'holding the American flag' for the school morning TV broadcast this past Monday. She wore her red, white, and blue (you all know how much she loves the 4th of July!), so it was just perfect. Her school is also celebrating 'Red Ribbon week' (to teach the students to say 'No' to drugs). Ironically, this morning, I asked her what she has been learning about drugs, and she got a sad look on her face. She said 'Mommy, I take drugs though- is that wrong?' I explained to her that 'drugs' can also be another name for medicine, and that it is okay to take medicine that doctors give you- but nothing else! Hopefully, that clarified it for her! I can only imagine what a 5 year old processes about all of

that!!!

The girls are looking forward to Halloween, and then a trip back up to Atlanta for Baby Will's christening. So, all is going well in the Koegel household. Right or wrong, we keep looking ahead to March 22nd as a light at the end of this tunnel. Sometimes it feels so close, and yet- on a day to day basis, treatment is very tiring (and I'm not even the patient!) She's a trooper...

Love to everyone, and we will keep you posted on her progress. Love, Rob, Kim, Taylor, and Alex

November 14, 2008

As I uploaded pictures to the website, I realized just how long it has been since the last update. Seeing all of the pictures and all that has been keeping Taylor busy made me smile though. Life has been filled with Halloween parades and parties at school, trick or treating, a trip to Atlanta for Baby Will's christening, field trips to the marine lab and football games. It is good for life to be filled with normal things....

Taylor had a trip to Gainesville last week, and while she was a little hesitant to go- she understood it was just a day trip, and that made it better. Her checkup went well- and her counts were all in acceptable ranges. They increased her daily chemo to nearly 100%. We will have her counts checked here locally next week, and the assumption is that she will be back up to 100% by then. Following her trip to clinic...it was the steroid stint for the month. I must admit that this one felt pretty tough. She had a good number of fits and frustration, and there seemed to be a lot of crying this time around. We also had to deal with our first call from school from the clinic (Taylor went there on Monday because she wasn't feeling good and wanted to come home). I got on the phone with her (recognizing that picking her up would be a bad precedent to set), and explained that her daddy and I would come have lunch with her and check in on her, but that she didn't have a fever and she wasn't sick, and that she would be just fine. She said "Okay, Mommy" and then I explained to the nurse that we appreciated the call, and that I would be there to have lunch with her and check on her. I was so appreciative of Taylor's teacher's support as well. Mrs. Shaw reminded me that it is important to keep Taylor in her day to day structure, and that sending her to school is the right thing to do. She is such a great lady! And Taylor just adores her....Well, Taylor made it through the school day, and then they had Veterans' Day off from school (which was timely), so by Wednesday- she was off of her steroids, and she felt a lot better. Getting to school the rest of the week has not been an issue!

So, we just continue to take it day by day- looking ahead to March 22, 2009 for that last dose of chemotherapy. I just hug her tight and hate that she has to go through all of this. Thank you again for all of your kind words and wishes though. We know there is a reason for all of this.....and her strength continues to amaze me every day. I will take some more time to update in the next week....Love to all....

Love, Rob, Kim, Taylor, and Alex

November 28, 2008

We hope everyone had a Happy Thanksgiving yesterday! We definitely had a lot to be thankful for in the Koegel household, and counted those blessings over and over again...

For the most part, we had a relaxing day. Rob was on shift until around 6 p.m., so we had planned for a later dinner (which is kinda nice actually- it gives you a good bit of the day to relax before the big dinner! Grandma and Grandpa were hosting dinner, so the girls and I headed over early in the morning to make brunch, watch the Macy's Day parade....and just relax. It was too cute- because when Grandma opened the door- Taylor had her pilgrim hat on and Alex wore Taylor's Indian headset (Taylor had made both of them this past week at school). Both of the girls were very excited about Thanksgiving...The girls helped Grandpa put up the Christmas lights and had fun playing with Alex's new kitchen set that we surprised her with as an early birthday gift (She turned 3 today!!!) Even though everyone was having a great time, and Taylor had a good bit of energy, I had happened to notice that Taylor's appetite hadn't been very big throughout the day- and I took her temp around 3 p.m. and it was at 101 degrees. My stomach dropped- as a temp over 100.4 degrees means a trip to the hospital for blood work and most likely an admit of at least 48 hours and IV antibiotics. My heart just broke for her. I knew she wanted to stay and have Thanksgiving dinner, but there really wasn't a choice. I took her up to the fire station to see Rob, and sadly the thermometer still read the same-I'm not sure what I expected- for it to be different or something? We coordinated with Shands, and were able to take her to the emergency room here in Tallahassee. She was a trooper- not real excited about having to go do all of this on Thanksgiving- but she really did a great job with everything. She had a chest x-ray, bloodwork, a strep test, and some other uncomfortable tests...including the need for the nurse to put a catheter in for a urine specimen. Not a tear the entire time we were there....she just kept telling us that she wanted to go home to Grandma's and enjoy dinner as a family. I told her that we just had to see what the test results looked like, and that there was a chance we could still make it home for dinner tonight....and that if we didn't- I'm sure Grandma, Aunt Debbie, and Alex would bring dinner to us. While we waited for the news- Grandpa kept her laughing by blowing up 'glove' balloons and playing catch with them. Daddy came as soon as he got off shift, and kept the laughing going too. We can't say enough about the TMH staff. They treated her like a princess- and got through all of the labs as fast as possible. Miss Susie even came down from the Pediatric unit to help by accessing Taylor's port (her buddy). It was giving us some trouble at first-but Miss Susie reassessed her and got the blood draw without issue. When the results came back- her chest x-ray was clear (i.e., no pneumonia!!!) and her counts were over 2000. Needless to say, we were thrilled as that meant there was a chance we were going home last night! The doctor explained that her white blood cells had a 'left shift.' (I had never heard of this before). He explained that a left shift indicates a bacterial infection and that a right shift indicates a viral infection. Whatever the cause- he wanted to give IV antibiotics as a precaution last night before sending her home....and then she started her weekly dose of Septra today (which is an antibiotic she takes each week to help ward off infections). So, all in all- the news was great. We got home to Grandma's around 10 p.m., and had a full Thanksgiving dinner. Taylor fought to keep her eyes open, but she had something to eat and was so happy. She snuggled up on the couch with Grandma, and we told her that we'd wake her up in a couple of hours for her chemo meds. She was okay with that.

Today, we headed out to have brunch with Grandma, Grandpa and Aunt Debbie and to celebrate Alex's 3rd birthday. Santa was at the restaurant- so the girls were pretty excited (although Alex wouldn't get too close to him!)

There are some Ariel cupcakes that we were going to have last night that we saved for tonight....Alex is pretty excited about them. It's just been a nice day spent together as a family. It's pretty rainy here right now, so we are just inside with a fire on and the porch doors open listening to the rain (and watching football....) Lots to cheer for this weekend- Go Tigers and Go Seminoles!!!

So, lots to feel thankful for....Taylor is resting right now, and we are just now looking ahead to her trip to Gainesville this coming week. She'll have her overnight visit for her spinal chemo and checkup, and then back home for lots of fun holiday activities. We'll keep everyone posted on her progress. Love to all...Love, Rob, Kim, Taylor, and Alex

December 6, 2008

Taylor had a great trip to Gainesville this week. It was a 2 day visit, and we were so happy that she didn't seem as anxious this time about having to stay overnight. The past 6 months have been quite a battle with trips to clinic- but this trip went very smoothly. Her ANC was over 1600, and her hematocrit and hemoglobin were at acceptable levels too. Her platelets were back up over 200 which was nice to see. It's funny- because my frame of reference is very limited about all of these numbers- except to know that there was a time when we were hoping to get her platelets up to 30 so she didn't have to continue transfusions.....but regardless, the past 2 years just feel like a crash course in medical stuff and I'll just try to explain her results the best I can!

She had her lumbar puncture (her spinal chemo) on Friday morning, and Rob said she even waved to him when they rolled her out of the Pre-Op area back to the operating room. Her strength continues to amaze us- or maybe the better phrase is inspire us...Rob and Taylor got back to Tallahassee yesterday afternoon and then surprised Alex and Mommy by getting a bunch of Christmas decorating done! I got home last night, and the tree was up....and then the girls and I put ornaments on it last night. It is always cute to me to watch the girls hang ornaments- if they could- they would put 20 ornaments on the same branch because it is the "perfect spot Mommy!"

We will push through another steroid stint this weekend, but we have a good bit going on (hopefully some good distractions). The girls, Grandma and I are headed to "The Nutcracker" ballet this morning and then there is the downtown Christmas festival tonight (with a parade and lots of lights....) So, we'll continue to try and find distractions that take her mind off of all of this. Ironically, I think Taylor is slightly happy about the steroid stint this time around- because it helps to clear up the skin issues she has been experiencing with the chemo. The Decadron seems to clear it up within a day- so I guess you take the good with the bad. I have to remember that she is getting

older- and that young ladies become very aware of their appearance at an early age....she hates that the redness on her face makes her look different, so we are trying to be diligent with applying cream to minimize the redness. I just remind myself that it is short term, and that while we continue to hear that the skin issues may increase for the first couple of months after she finishes chemo- we will get through that too. She has been through various things / side effects with treatment- several of them much worse, and she'll get through this part too. The only other challenge she seems to be having right now is low sugar on some mornings- it comes and goes- there doesn't seem to be a logic to when it happens. So, we push through that as well....Alex even recognizes everything going on and tells Rob and me "GO GET THE JUICE !!! I'LL GET THE TOWEL!!!"

So- all is going as best as can be expected in the Koegel household. Life feels busy, and while we count down the days until the end of Taylor's chemo, we also have come to realize that there is no end to any of this. Her end of treatment date is a milestone, but it is also just the beginning of a new phase- and the reality of seeing if her body is able to ward the cancer off without the drugs. For the longest time, we had planned to have a big party in March- now, I think we are reevaluating....We think it is still a good idea to recognize it, but we also don't want to confuse Taylor. All of this is still very much an unknown... because there will still be some medicine to take for at least 6 months or so (most likely antibiotics while her immune system rebuilds itself)....there will still be lumbar punctures (without the chemo, but to check that the spinal fluid is clear of cancer)....and there will continue to be monthly trips to clinic and regular visits for bloodwork for the foreseeable future. So for now- we've planned a trip to Disney World next Spring and told her that we will have popcorn and snacks late at night (because she won't have to cut off food / drink due to late night medicine)! She's pretty excited about that! As March gets closer, maybe we'll have other ideas too, but we will recognize it as a milestone. More than anything, we want this to be the end of everything that deals with Leukemia- and it might be....and if it's not, well then we'll take that as it comes too. Having said that, everything inside of me tells me it is going to be okay, and it will be, and she will be fine. I'm sure that every parent of a child with cancer goes through these roller coaster emotions, and you just have to turn it over to God and his divine plan. If nothing else, I remind myself every day to keep work and life and other things bugging me in check...and to just enjoy the wonderful things that life brings us each day...The holidays are also a great way of reinforcing that. So with that perspective in mind- I am headed off to get breakfast ready for my hungry crew and get them ready for the Nutcracker ballet this morning- they are so excited!!! Love to all, and thank you again for all of your love and support on this journey...

Love, Rob, Kim, Taylor, and Alex

December 30, 2008

Merry Christmas and Happy New Year to everyone! It is hard to believe that 2009 is just around the corner....

We had a wonderful Christmas- complete with Christmas morning here in Tallahassee, and then a trip to Port Saint Lucie in time for Christmas dinner. Taylor and Alex were both so excited about Christmas, and I really just loved soaking in all of their excitement about it all (setting out the cookies for Santa...getting to bed in time for him to

251

come....Taylor waking up at 3 a.m. and coming into our room to tell us that she was "sure that he had come already Mommy- can't we just quick check downstairs???") Taylor was thrilled that Santa brought her the items on her Christmas list- a hula hoop, a toy pony, and American Girl Doll clothes. Alex was thrilled with just about everything, especially her 'Fur-Real' dog that she named 'Fernando...'

In January 2007, when Taylor was diagnosed, 2009 seemed a forever away....and yet here we are. I am hopeful that it brings a much needed year of transition for us, and that we are able to overcome any fears that go along with the end of treatment. We'll just continue to take each day as it comes. March 22nd will be a very celebrated day, so it is hard to believe it is truly so close.

Taylor had her monthly visit to Shands yesterday. Her counts were a little lower than expected (ANC was 940), but her doctors were not concerned. The lower counts were most likely due to a cold she has been fighting, but everything was in acceptable ranges, so her daily chemo will continue at 100%. Many thanks to her doctors who allowed us to move up her appointment to yesterday (her appointment was supposed to be on January 1st, but clinic is closed that day). By having her appointment yesterday, it allowed us to start her steroid stint earlier so that she can battle out the stint while she is still on Christmas break. It also allowed me to take off a week from work over the holidays (when it is technically slower) to help her get through it. On this schedule, she'll be done with the stint and the side effects should subside prior to her going back to school next week. Alex also has school 3 days this week, so it gives us the opportunity to keep her in a structured environment (and away from Taylor) during the majority of the stint. That way, Alex doesn't have to be exposed to as many outbursts, and she can have her normal day to day activities with her friends at school.

I will share that we have been a bit nervous about Alex lately...she has been showing 'trends / behaviors' that Taylor exhibited about a month or so prior to her diagnosis a couple of years ago...complaining about being sleepy, regression of potty training at night, trouble getting over colds....I know that a lot of this could be explained away by a million reasons- including just being 3 years old. However, you can imagine our sensitivity to it. We've talked to our pediatrician as well as the doctors at Shands, and we did have Alex's blood counts done. Everything came back normal, but the change in behavior is continuing, so we did talk to Shands again yesterday. The bottom line is that we have read that siblings are 2-4 times more at risk for getting it; however, with the number of children diagnosed each year, the chances are still pretty low....Taylor's doctors explained that there is nothing we can do to prevent it- and that while it would be rare for it to happen, it could....and that if it did, we would know it when it happened....and that if it does happen, we'll get her counts checked and that's what will show it. So, we are hopeful that we are just overly sensitive to things right now, but we are also feeling like we are reliving scenarios from 2 years ago- so we want to pay close attention. If it did actually happen, we'll just take a deep breath and take the next step. It doesn't even seem it could be possible, so we try not to think about it more than we have to....

As we wrap up 2008, I just want to express our gratitude to all of you who follow Taylor's journey. We appreciate everything that folks have done to help us along the way- our families and friends have been amazing, and are there to help us at every turn. Thank you so much. Here's looking forward to a year filled with hope- for Taylor and for all of the children out there who are going through treatment, and for those that may get that news this year. Life is just so precious, and if there is one thing I wish for everyone in the upcoming year is that we all appreciate the little miracles that happen around us every day....hug your family tight, tell each other 'I love you' and don't let the small stuff get to you too much...it's just not that important.....

Love to all and Happy New Year!

Love, Rob, Kim, Taylor, and Alex

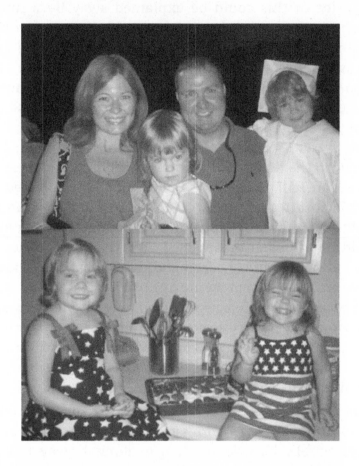

2009

I am happy to say that Christmas break wrapped up very nicely, including Taylor's steroid stint. While I'm sure it was not the way that Taylor preferred to spend the second half of her Christmas break, it is nice to know that she has had a couple of days for the side effects to leave her system, and that things are back to 'normal' in time for school to resume tomorrow.

While it doesn't seem right to ever wish time away, steroid stint weeks are times where I often do that. I just keep telling myself things like..."Okay, we're x% of the way through this stint...we're almost there...only 2 more days, etc." Since she wrapped up on Saturday, the residual effects seemed to be gone by yesterday evening, so today was really a nice 'Mommy / Taylor' day....which was nice to have before she went back to school. We had our nails painted, went to lunch at Boston Market (her favorite place ever....), and then spent time at the library this afternoon. I am embarrassed to say that she already had her library card (and I had to apply for one today)....but what a great place to spend the afternoon with your child- she absolutely loves the library! She came home with 7 books. So, after getting to spend some one on one time with my sweet girl...I am a bit sad that work and school will start again this week, but it will be good for us to get back to our routine too.

I've posted some pictures from the past few weeks- including some from Christmas, our trip to Port Saint Lucie / Ft. Pierce, and New Year's. There is also a great one of Taylor with her friends Cade and Jenna at the playground here in Tallahassee. These are 2 of her friends from pre-school that she hadn't seen in months. It was great for them to have some time to play together over the break! One of my favorite pictures is the picture of Taylor and Alex picking oranges at Grandma and Grandpa's house in Sarasota....(yes- there is still a house in Sarasota!) Taylor and Alex love that Grandma and Grandpa have a house here and a house in Sarasota, although I'm sure Grandma and Grandpa would love to sell it at some point! Someone told Grandpa that the picture of the girls is a great commercial for Publix- I thought that was pretty funny....Actually, it just reminds me of Debbie and I growing up in that house, and going outside to pick oranges in the winter time....when we were real little, I remember making fresh orange juice in the morning time with those oranges....as I'm sure every family from New Jersey did for at least the first 6 months after they moved to Florida!....lots of good memories at that house...

I wanted to say thank you to everyone who has checked in with us about Alex too....Things remain status quo, so that is a good thing for now. We do hope that we are just being overly sensitive, and that everything will be just fine. So, with that...things are going well in the Koegel household...we just continue to look forward to the new year and the hope that it brings. Thank you again to all who continue to follow Taylor's journey. Love to all....Love, Rob, Kim, Taylor, and Alex

January 14, 2009

I write this as we kick off the Relay for Life effort for Team Princess Taylor (http://main.acsevents.org/goto/teamprincesstaylor). I updated the Team Princess Taylor site last night, and I will admit that I cried most of the way through it. It is just a surreal experience to realize that your family is actually going through all of this...but you push through and you move on. The Relay is a very emotional experience, and it is hard to explain. You get your team together...you walk...you laugh, you cry, you bond...and you hope that the money you raise is truly making a difference- and it does. Taylor asked me last year why we relay, and I tried to break it down into simple terms for her. I explained that we relay to raise money to help the scientists buy more microscopes to study cancer germs. She understood that, and why we walk. She told me that she won't be scared to walk in the 'Survivor' lap this year. I told her that I would carry her the whole way if she wanted me to...

Thank you to everyone who signed up today for the team. Everyone's team site was inspiring....Grandma and Grandpa relay for so many loved ones...Lori is relaying for various loved ones, and specifically a mom who passed away this past weekend in Tallahassee from breast cancer...Angie continues to relay for Sarah-there are so many stories. Aunt Debbie's site made me tear up- as I realized how much we share as a part of Taylor's Caring Bridge site- here is an excerpt from Debbie's site:

"I relay because I never want another child to have steroid weekends, to lose their hair, to have to have spinal taps, to have to have bone marrow biopsies, to have ports accessed, to be neutropenic, to have to have daily chemo, to know that you have to wait 2 hours after eating dinner to take 6MP, to have to go get counts checked, and to know what all the above mentioned means..."

Thank you Aunt Debbie, and thank you to everyone who has signed up for the Relay...and thank you to all of you who continue to follow us on this journey. I try so hard to never call it a battle- because that would imply that it could be lost. I know that sounds a little extreme, but I read that early on in Taylor's diagnosis, and it has stuck with me. I will never allow myself to believe that she or any other child 'loses this battle....' All of these children are fighters...

As an update- we had Taylor's counts checked yesterday (as

she has been fighting a yucky cough). Thankfully her counts came back at good levels...ANC was over 900, her hematocrit and hemoglobin were at acceptable levels, and her platelets were over 200. It was a sigh of relief, and we were happy to not have to make a decision to keep her out of school. Consistency and schedule are good for all of us- and it breaks my heart to have to pull her out of school and her activities.

Thank you again to all of you. You have continued to follow our every update and roller coaster of emotions....and we are so appreciative.

Love, Rob, Kim, Taylor, and Alex

January 19, 2009

It has been a day of reflection, as we look back to 2 years ago today, and the day that this journey started for Taylor and our family. January 19th, 2007 was the day we went into our pediatrician's office (after a late night visit to urgent care the night before, complete with lab work), and heard the news that the pediatrician feared that Taylor had Leukemia. His recommendation was to transport her to Shands for assessment of the situation, but only after we took her to our local hospital to confirm she was stable enough for the two-hour ambulance trip to Gainesville....

I remember every moment of that day- I can still tell you what Taylor was wearing- (her little Carlos and Charlie's shirt from Aruba actually...)...I can tell you the sick feeling as I looked at Rob, as the nurses in the doctor's office hugged me and told me "We are here for you no matter what you need..." And all I wanted to say was "I need someone to tell me my child is going to live!" Of course, I was too choked up and in shock to say much of anything other than "What do we do now?" And then the roller coaster started...

But here we are! Taylor has 62 days of chemotherapy left. That translates into 1 more lumbar puncture, 2 more steroid stints, 62 days of 6MP, 8 doses of Methotrexate...and a good bit of Zofran along the way...but she is going to hit that milestone with flying colors. In her mind, she is just excited about having some popcorn to eat in the evenings soon....Yes, there will be antibiotics for at least 6 months, a surgery to remove her port at some point, and ongoing visits to Shands for checkups for years to come- but there will be popcorn at night (at least some nights!)

We had dinner at Grandma and Grandpa's house tonight, and I was just watching my energetic little 5 year old dance around the family room with her sister...and talking about how she is going to gymnastics and dance this week...It is such a stark contrast to 2 years ago when she was weak and in need of blood and platelet transfusions and lying in a hospital bed. I remember going to sleep at the hotel in Gainesville 2 years ago tonight (Rob was at the hospital with Taylor and I'm pretty sure 10 people couldn't have pulled him away from her). I remember waking up the next morning, realizing I was in a hotel in Gainesville, and closing my eyes again to cry...as I realized this was all happening- it wasn't just a bad dream. I thank God every day for the knowledge, medicine and tools that her doctors have and the time we have continued to have with Taylor. Even as I reread through journal entries, there are times when I feel that I do dwell on everything that has happened over the past 2 years- but in all honesty, it is hard not to! I try not to think of it as dwelling as much as I try to think of it as remembering where everything started and how far Taylor has come and we have continued to grow as a family during this time...and I see how such an awful thing has impacted us in so many positive ways too! We have been blessed by the generosity of friends and family, and these are all very positive things for the girls to understand....how to help others in a time of need...how to give back to their community- these are all very positive. Part of me would be happy to take these lessons and move on and never have to think about cancer again- but that is not realistic (and not in my hands either).

So with this long entry tonight, I just want to say thank you to everyone again. Thank you for so many things- your continued support of our family, for helping to increase awareness about childhood cancer...for everything. We will take pictures of our little gymnast this week (as she is very excited about this new endeavor...), and we will keep everyone posted on the weeks to come. Love to all...

Love, Rob, Kim, Taylor, and Alex

January 29, 2009

Taylor made her monthly trip to Shands today, and her checkup went well. Her ANC was over 1700, and her white blood count, hematocrit and hemoglobin were at acceptable levels too. It is hard to believe that there are only 2 more trips to clinic that include IV and spinal chemo. Spread across those 2 more trips are 52 days left of her daily chemo....it's just hard to comprehend that she will soon be done with this daily regimen. The monthly trips will continue, and Rob was able to ask the doctors some additional questions about what else will follow. I give the doctors a lot of credit for giving us things in logical 'chunks...' (i.e., there is only so much you can process at one time!) So, it looks like the next steps are that she will (1) make her February trip to Shands for her checkup and quarterly lumbar puncture (with spinal chemo), (2) take her last dose of chemo on March 22nd and then (3) make a trip to Shands on March 26th for a bone marrow biopsy and to have a lumbar puncture (without spinal chemo though....just to pull spinal fluid to confirm it is clear of cancer). At some point, the doctors will do a surgery to remove her port...(we're assuming approximately 6 months post end of treatment date), and then we just continue to take one day at a time...Wow! Life is good...

So, other than processing the milestones that are coming-things have been going well in our household. Taylor and Alex continue to be busy with dance classes, and now Taylor has started gymnastics too. She absolutely loves it, and we continue to appreciate how all of this exercise must be good to keep her muscles strong...

Taylor had her first school project this week- it was called 'All About Me.' Each child had a specific week over the school year for their poster, and the week of January 26th was Taylor's week. The project was interesting, as Rob and I were both very conscious about not weighing in about what he and I would include as part of the poster- we wanted to defer to Taylor to see how she would explain 'All About Me...' It was insightful. While it was a long process for her to look through digital pictures from the past 5 years, she knew in her mind what she wanted...she explained to me "No baby pictures Mommy- only big kid pictures...."...and then she narrowed that down to "only having pictures from Kindergarten on"- and while she didn't specifically say this- nothing was specific to anything that had to do with cancer. There were several pictures of her and Alex, several pictures of her doing gymnastics and dance, and pictures of Aruba and DisneyWorld. She put lots of stickers on her poster, and chose to bring in her 'American Girl Doll' to share with her class. I guess the key thing Rob and I took from this whole project was a valuable point for Rob and I to understand: Taylor doesn't define herself as someone with cancer....Instead, she sees herself as a big sister, a daughter, a gymnast and a dancer...and just a kid. The flip side is that we wouldn't have had a concern if she did have various pictures of her cancer journey on her poster because it is part of who she is and it has contributed to the strong person she is- but she's not ready to (or doesn't want to) highlight that at this point in her life. There may be more to that, and someday she may be more comfortable talking about some of it- but for now, we talk about it with her when she wants to talk about it....and we listen to her when she says she doesn't want to focus on it- we try to be sensitive to what she tells us. We'll see what the coming months bring and just continue to support her! The good news is that she was proud of her school project and was so excited to talk about it this week.

She was in good spirits tonight, and we are looking ahead to her second to last steroid stint this weekend. We will push through, and we will remember that the Decadron is just finishing up its job of blowing up those bad cells. We will keep everyone posted on her progress, and we thank you again for you continued support and prayers.

Love to all...Love, Rob, Kim, Taylor, and Alex

February 8, 2009

Last night was a big date night for Taylor and Rob....as they headed out to the Daddy / Daughter dance! Some of you may remember the big outing last year...and the Daddies surprising 5 little girls with a limo to go to the dance...well, the Daddies didn't disappoint this year either! The girls had a great time, and I've heard there was a lot of dancing going on!!! As you'll see from the pictures, there were 5 little princesses pretty excited about the big night, and these were just my attempt at some pictures. Many thanks to Mr. Ray who came by to take some really fancy pictures...we can't wait to see them!

While Taylor and Rob were out on their big date, Alex and Mommy spent some fun time together too....heading to dinner of her choice (Chick-Fil-A) and Build A Bear to pick out some bear outfits. Alex will head to the dance next year...and Rob will be a lucky guy there with 2 dates, but we figured we'd wait until she was 4 years old, and can "hang out" as late as the rest of the gang did last night.

All continues to go well in the Koegel household- I can't quite explain the anticipation of knowing that her chemo is wrapping up in 43 days (maybe you can sense it....with me counting and all...). Finishing up her steroid stint this past week, and realizing that there is only 1 stint left was just crazy. Rob and I were talking last night about what comes next and are curious about whether we have a "roadmap" from the doctors for this next phase (as they have provided us for each phase in the past)....although we're not sure what a map for this "phase" would look like? How do you have a phase for "forever?" Most likely there is a series of next steps, including the lumbar puncture (LP) on March 26th. Rob explained that the doctors told him they do that LP and bone marrow biopsy to make sure there are no cancer cells left. When he said that, it was a slight wake up call for me, as I am assuming there have been none for a long time. I'll continue to think that way because there is really no reason to think any other way right now. (And we would drive ourselves crazy trying to imagine any other scenario at the moment).

Thank you to everyone who has been asking about the Relay for Life Team: Team Princess Taylor (http://main.acsevents.org/goto/teamprincesstaylor). The event is on May 1st this year (in Tallahassee), and we are so proud that the team has already raised nearly $1200! Thank you to everyone for your ongoing support of such an important cause!!! Consider walking with us here- or in your hometown. It is truly an impactful event to be involved with...I know it has been for us.

Well, I'll leave everyone with a funny story from our house recently. Taylor and Alex have some 'new' favorite songs....they are becoming big Jimmy Buffet fans...so, look for a couple little girls singing 'Fins' as we drive down the road these days, complete with all of the shark hand motions. Taylor told Rob the other day that she and Alex are parrotheads now...after he finished laughing, he asked her where she had heard that...and she told him that Mommy explained that it was a word for people who really liked Jimmy Buffet songs....so, there are now officially 2 more parrotheads out there :)

So, we will keep everyone posted on her progress and the

next steps (as we understand them better!) Love to all, and thank you again for your prayers for Taylor. It really means a lot.

Love, Rob, Kim, Taylor, and Alex

February 23, 2009

The days until the end of Taylor's chemotherapy continue to count down....27 to go. The mini-milestones are starting to happen....Taylor was at clinic today and had her LAST dose of Vincristine....tomorrow morning, she will have her LAST dose of spinal chemotherapy....and tomorrow begins her LAST steroid stint. Yes, you read that right. There will be some champagne poured this weekend....

Taylor had a good visit to clinic today- her ANC was over 1400 (with white blood cell, hematocrit, hemoglobin, and platelet counts all at acceptable levels). She wasn't anxious about having her buddy accessed, and she had a nice dinner date with her Daddy at Subway after wrapping up at clinic. I had to laugh / cringe (whatever the best term would be)... because the doctors increased her dosage of Decadron and 6-MP today (to account for her current weight). I told Rob- "It's her last steroid stint- I guess we're just going to go out with a bang!" At least we are trying to keep our sense of humor through some of this...

Rob said she was having a great trip to Gainesville overall....Taylor brought 'Chutes and Ladders' with her for the hotel tonight- I'm sure there is a crazy board game tournament going on down in Gainesville tonight! (She's got a mean game face for Chutes and Ladders....Just ask Aunt Debbie, Miss KC, and Miss Leigh!)

We worked with her doctors to have her clinic visit and lumbar puncture scheduled a little early this week. She was originally supposed to head down this Thursday / Friday- but she has her first school program on Friday morning, and she is so excited about it. When Rob and I realized the date, we reached out to Shands to understand if there was a possibility to shift the date by a day or two (understanding that her chemotherapy is the first priority, but wanted to at least see if there was an option). Her doctors explained that they could shift it by a few days, and gave us the option of Monday / Tuesday.....We talked to Taylor about it, and she was thrilled that she would be able to be at school for her show. I'm glad that even in the midst of all of this- we can still help her be a kid....

As I type this, it is hard to believe that we are so close to March 22, 2009- a date that we have been marching toward for what feels like an eternity- yet it is so close. I had lunch with my friend Angie today, and she asked me how I felt about March 22nd approaching, and the best word I could find was "anxious." I'm happy, and believe me- Rob and I are happy that her little body will get a break from daily doses of chemo- but you do wonder what comes next. My heart tells me to celebrate! I want to shout out loud that Taylor is done! And then there is the practical side of me that says "Don't confuse her- just let everything play out...." I'm sure in the days / weeks / months to come- things will become more clear....our family will begin to adjust....and we will start to feel more comfortable that the cancer will stay away, and we'll know better what and how to feel.

Before signing off tonight, I just want to continue to say Thank You to everyone. You've continued to follow Taylor's journey- through all of the ups and downs- and your prayers continue to surround our family with support. We also appreciate the continuous offers for help from friends and family- I thank God every day that we have family so close- helping to pick up the kids....dinners...making sure Alex has special attention and a place to stay when "fussy medicine" makes life crazy at our house...we are forever grateful.

We'll keep everyone posted on the weeks to come. Love to all....Love, Rob, Kim, Taylor, and Alex

March 2, 2009

Just a quick update- but a happy one- as the final steroid stint is now complete! Her last dose was Saturday night, and I'm not sure what I exactly expected.....fireworks? angels singing? something? Instead- Taylor took her medicine, went to bed, and slept soundly- a very nice end to all of this. Rob was kind enough to leave the empty bottle on the counter for me....he knew I wanted to do something with it- throw it against the wall, run over it with the car (throwing it away just seemed too kind). But in the end, that's exactly what we did- just threw the bottle away and moved on- just like Taylor seems to do with all of this. When we told her it was her last dose of 'Decadron,' she just rolled her eyes and said "I know, I know- I'm done soon- can we read my book now?" Good lessons to learn from kids- don't dwell :)

So- we pushed through the lasting side effects yesterday (attitude and big appetite), but she woke up a refreshed person this morning, and ready to go to school. Many thanks to Grandma and Grandpa for letting Alex camp out this weekend at their house while we pushed through the last couple of days.

So, one more mini-milestone down- 20 days of chemo to go! Love to all, and we'll keep you posted on the upcoming weeks! Love, Rob, Kim, Taylor, and Alex

March 17, 2009

So here we are on Tuesday...with only 5 doses of chemo left to give. I was watching Taylor tonight at Gymnastics, and as I looked at the determination on her face (she is like a machine when she goes after her somersaults and backwards rolls)- I just started to tear up. And- by the way- I bet I was the only parent in the place thinking "Next week, we can surprise her with a treat other than water after gymnastics.... something (dare I consider it) with citric acid?" I know- that may sound foreign to a lot of you- but just ask Taylor- she knows she can't have citric acid at night- it may block the absorption of her chemo meds.....Yes, I know- we have tried to follow the letter of the law with this stuff- but we don't want to take any chances. But back to the fact that there are only 5 days left of chemo- we are so excited for her- excited that her body will get a rest from all of this medicine, and excited that she reaches yet another mini-milestone with treatment.

With regard to milestones, I started going through pictures this week of the last 27 months of treatment. I'll post a few each night as we get closer to Sunday- I posted some from December 2006 - July 2007 tonight....(and then some current pictures from this past weekend from a fun family visit!) As I look at these pictures, there are definitely some teary moments- but if you can believe it, some laughter too (thinking back to some of the trips to the butterfly garden and picnics at the park). Most importantly, I am reminded of the continuous progress she has made. I also watch Alex growing up in these pictures, and I am reminded that this has consumed her life as well. While I do hope that some of the scary and sad memories fade for both kids, I'm sure that there are parts of their character that have been forever molded as a result of this. I look at Alex and see a compassionate 3-year-old- a kid who will run to get a towel for her sister when she is throwing up in the morning. I also see a 3-year-old that probably knows a little too much detail about meds...(i.e., she feeds her baby dolls pretend Septra and 6-MP)....but I'm sure over time, that may fade. What I love to see is the bond that they have as sisters- even though it feels like they fight like cats and dogs sometimes- there is an unbreakable bond between them.

So....looking ahead: After that final, ceremonial last dose of medicine this coming Sunday (yes, listen for the cheers, the tears- whatever...probably sometime between 8 - 9 p.m. on March 22nd)....we will head down to Gainesville next Thursday and Friday. Taylor will have a bone marrow biopsy and they will draw some spinal fluid to confirm that both the marrow and the spinal fluid are clear of any cancer. That will be the first sigh of relief. Following those results, she will continue her monthly visits to Shands for checkups (but no chemo). In 6 months, she'll have her port out....but let's not get too far ahead of ourselves. If this journey has taught us anything, it is to take one step at a time- and appreciate every day that God gives us with our loved ones.

As we wrap this phase in Taylor's treatment, it is also timely for our continued focus on Relay for Life activities (coming up May 1st). Team Princess Taylor (http://main.acsevents.org/goto/teamprincesstaylor)continues to raise money to support such an important cause. Rob and I invite you to join our team- come walk with us...or take the opportunity to walk at a local Relay- it is truly a time of reflection...and while it will be a time for celebration for us as well (as we think about the amazing strides made in research, and the time it has provided us with Taylor), there is still so much more work to be done. We'd love to have you on the team....

Thanks for reading the long post tonight- as my friend Kim said in a message today "I can only imagine the range of emotions you're going through this week...." So- tonight, I took the time to share some of them. Believe me, it would take another couple of pages to get them all on paper :) Love to all, and we will keep everyone posted on this week, next week, and the months to come. Love, Rob, Kim, Taylor, and Alex

March 23, 2009

A quick update (and a promise to update later tonight, as it has been a busy week with lots to journal about)-but this was an event that we could not let pass without an update!!!

Taylor took her last dose of chemo last night!

It was a sigh of relief, an evening for reflection, the "end of an era" as one of my friends put it last night- but most importantly- the completion of another milestone in her treatment. I think tonight will be the more interesting night, as there will be no 6-MP to give- it will definitely feel weird! Just to make sure there was no confusion, I immediately threw away anything that resembled a chemo drug last night :) There were some silent screams of joy when I saw Rob come up the stairs with her last dose....and I was almost laughing as I did the "double check" of the doses...I asked him "Do you have the 6-MP, the Zofran, and the Septra?" He reminded me that he's been doing this for 27 months...and he was pretty sure he had it straight. I was reading books with Alex at the time, and she just started clapping her hands and said "Yea Mommy, we're all done with medicine!"

We look ahead now to Thursday and Friday of this week for her bone marrow biopsy and checking of spinal fluid (to make sure there are no signs of cancer).

Thank you, thank you, thank you again for your continued support through this. We will keep you posted on her procedures this week, and we are just so thankful for how the past 27 months have progressed. It has been quite a journey, and while there is still more to go- we're happy to wrap up this chapter.

Love to all...Love, Rob, Kim, Taylor, and Alex

March 27, 2009

This is a picture of Taylor 'ringing the bell' at clinic yesterday (to signify the end of her chemo!) It was a pretty emotional moment- and very special actually- all of the doctors, nurses, PAs, etc. that have been there with us through all of this surprised her by coming into the room and singing the following: (to the tune of the Oscar Mayer song):

Our patient has the cutest smile, it's S-M-I-LE
Our patient has the sweetest heart, it's H-E-A-R-T
We love to see you every day, but if you ask us now we'll

say.......

Pack your bags, get out the door, cause you don't have chemo anymore!

They also gave her a trophy and a certificate for her bravery during treatment. I will admit I was pretty choked up during the whole thing...Taylor actually shies away from a lot of attention....and she was a little shy while they sang yesterday, but later on in the car- she kept asking me to sing the song again.

The trip to clinic yesterday was definitely different than previous trips- for one- there was no chemo! She had labs done- her ANC was over 2400 with some of her labs even being in "normal" ranges. Amazing! She also had a routine checkup with the doctors, and we discussed what comes next. She'll take Septra for the next 6 months to help her counts continue to strengthen, and we'll continue to come down for monthly visits for labs and for the doctors to see her in person. That will go on for at least 1 year, and then the frequency between visits may lessen...Assuming all goes well today with her bone marrow biopsy and spinal fluid check (i.e., no sign of cancer still present), her doctors would actually like to schedule the consult with the pediatric surgeon for next month when we're at Shands for her monthly visit. The consult will be for taking her port out....maybe within the next 2 months. It was a lot to process, but signifies that she continues to move through all of this.

The doctors asked me if I had any questions, and of course my first one was "How quickly will we know the results of the bone marrow biopsy?" They told me it will most likely be Monday or Tuesday. I made sure they had every contact number possible.

There is so much to journal about- so much that has gone on in the past couple of weeks, and I have such good intent to update every night, and I will find a way to get it all out there- it has just been a really long week. It has actually been a week of varied emotions- thrilled that Taylor is done with chemo, funny at moments (Taylor realizing...and us too...that it wasn't the end of the world that we didn't fit dinner in BEFORE dance class on Wednesday night....we didn't have medicine dictating our schedule that night), and then yesterday an emotion snuck up on me on the way to clinic- I felt like I was going to get sick. Yeah- that doesn't sound so pleasant, but as I got off at Archer (the interstate exit for clinic), and made our way toward Shands, I literally felt sick. It lasted through her appointment yesterday, and even into dinner and our trip to the mall. I don't want to say I'm scared of what is next- it is just an unknown. There has been a roadmap for all of treatment- there isn't one now. There have been medicines to keep the cancer at bay- those are done now too. But (I remind myself), that is all part of how this works. She is a strong little girl, and we will continue to pray that she stays healthy. I told Rob the other night that I continue to pray that God's will is done- but selfishly, I also pray that it is to keep Taylor healthy....and if for some reason the outcome is different...then I pray to be able to reconcile the difference and understand it the best that I can. My friend Kathryn has an amazing way of sending "just the right emails at just the right time" over the past 27 months...and I hadn't had a chance to talk through all of this with her yet- and then this email arrived yesterday:

"The will of God will never take you where the grace of God will not protect you."

Needless to say- it was perfect timing....something that helped to ease my mind when I read it again last night at the hotel.

Her doctors also explained to me yesterday that if the cancer is going to come back, it will most likely come back quick....and that she has done well during treatment- being in remission now for over 2 years! Dr. Slayton also upped her prognosis by another couple of percentage points....he said that treatment is now showing an 85% chance that she will never relapse. That was a nice thing to hear before leaving clinic....So, with that in mind, we will continue to move forward...and everything in me tells me that things will go just fine this morning. Taylor is a bit anxious for some reason- she did not sleep well tonight. She heard my cell phone buzz in the middle of the night, and she sprung out of bed saying "Is it time? Is that the hotel calling us to wake up?" I told her "no sweetie, it's okay, go back to sleep...." She wanted me to just snuggle with her, and it took her awhile, but eventually she went back to sleep.

Thank you again for your prayers for Taylor. We will keep everyone posted on the outcome of her biopsy, and the weeks / months to come. Our family is truly blessed to have all of you with us on this journey. Love to all...

Love, Rob, Kim, Taylor, and Alex

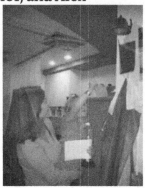

March 31, 2009

Our internet connection has been touch and go tonight- so just a short, but great update....here is the report from Shands today:

"There is no pathological evidence of Acute Lymphoblastic Leukemia cells from the biopsy..." Translation: There is no sign of cancer!!!

Rob put it best- "We used to say Taylor 'has' Leukemia...Now we say she 'had' Leukemia..."

Love to all, and promises to update more shortly! Love, Rob, Kim, Taylor, and Alex

April 1, 2009

The roller coaster continued a bit today....we got a follow-up call from Shands. The good news is that the outcome still stands about their assessment of "no pathological evidence of Leukemia cells..." The part that was a little concerning was that Taylor's doctor called to tell us that they did identify a clump of abnormal cells in the sample. Thankfully, he went on to explain that they sometimes see this (and have seen this a good bit in the past year) as part of the post treatment biopsies....and that typically a follow-up biopsy done 1 month later shows no sign of the abnormal cells. Another thing to be thankful for was that Rob was the one on the phone with the doctor....I don't think I would have handled the news as calmly as he did. He really is a rock through all of this. He asked Dr. Slayton (on a scale of 1-10) how worried we should be, and Dr. Slayton said "1." We have trusted this man with our daughter for the past 27 months, and we have no reason to doubt his assessment now....So, Taylor will have another biopsy at the end of April with the hope that all of it comes back clear.

I will admit that I did go through a range of emotions today-one being a bit of anger and frustration as to why the doctor who called yesterday seemed to not have the whole picture when she gave me the news....however, after calming down-I realized that it really didn't matter....it is what it is....AND Rob reminded me that the cancer is still gone. I just question what 'abnormal' means? It feels like such a generic term. Does it mean pre-cancerous cells? Does it just mean cells impacted by high intensity chemo?

After we had some time to process this today, we have a ton of questions for Dr. Slayton....how do the doctors track this? Is this something new they are seeing? Do they think it is abnormal cells due to the intensity of the chemo? (and then as the body chemistry normalizes....the cells disappear which is why the next biopsy is fine?) So many questions- but still trying to focus on the happiness we felt yesterday and should continue to feel about there being no trace of Leukemia cells.

The will of God will not lead us where the grace of God will not protect us....I had to remind myself of that today too.

Other than the unsettling phone call today, our 'celebration' vacation week has been fun. The girls have had a blast in Orlando, and have spent time at Disney with Grandma, Grandpa, Aunt Debbie, and Luke....and then down to Port Saint Lucie today to spend time with Gammy, Aunt Kathy, Uncle Jack, and Aunt Gwen....it has been a good week of memories (including Taylor's first rides on Thunder Mountain and Space Mountain!) We knew she was brave..... :) Ironically, my camera decided to go on the fritz right before lunch at the castle yesterday with Cinderella and the princesses....but I don't think any of us need pictures to remember those memories- they are etched in my mind. Taylor and Alex were smiling from ear to ear (and we tried to get some pics on the cell phones too....just in case one might turn out!)

So, I'll wrap up now, and get some much-needed sleep. Rob and I really feel exhausted- emotionally....everything. None of this will ever truly be over, but hopefully next month will bring us a little closer to closure. The results this week were a huge step, and we don't want to forget that- and we will continue to have faith that all will be fine.

Love to all...Love, Rob, Kim, Taylor, and Alex

April 2, 2009

Just a quick update to say that we spoke with Dr. Slayton again today. I had put a call into him yesterday to talk about some of the questions Rob and I had....he called this morning, and reassured me that "abnormal" does not mean pre-cancerous and that he has no reason to think these "abnormal" cells are Leukemia. He did say (and understandably so) that he just wants to be vigilant about doing another biopsy....because there is always a small chance that this could be something brewing, and he wants to be on top of it. So- while I would love for him to give me some 100% comfort level that every-thing is fine- I know that is not realistic- so we will just take it day by day....hour by hour....until we get to the next biopsy and the results.

Vacation continues to be great....I tried as much as possible to put this stuff out of my mind today and enjoy the fact that we are on vacation. We spent time at the pool and play-ing outside, and the girls are resting now before we head to dinner.

Love to all- and we will keep you posted on the weeks to come...Love, Rob, Kim, Taylor, and Alex

April 7, 2009

Back to work and school! The kids were a bit slow getting out of bed yesterday (as were Mommy and Daddy too!), but all went well- and both of the girls had great days at school. I took time yesterday to just be thankful for all of the great times we had this past week...To see Taylor swimming, run-ning, playing- to not have the week dictated by medicine or having to time dinner "just right" so that she could take her medicine before bedtime....it was all just such a blessing.

I will admit that I have been surprised at how easy it has been to adjust to life without medicine. It really hasn't been a second thought now, and I am happy about that...nothing to dwell on, just looking ahead to getting that next biopsy and the results. I am hoping that brings a bit more closure to all of this.

I did want to let everyone know that Grandma and Grandpa have a contract on the house in Sarasota! It happened the same week that Taylor was done with her medicine. The girls and I made one last trip to see the house (a quick trip)- but one that I wanted to make. I walked through the house one last time, remembering all of the amazing memories from the past 30+ years there....it was a bittersweet visit- so happy that Mom and Dad are here in Tallahassee with us (and grateful for all of their help), but sad to be selling the house too. Taylor said that she's pretty sure that the new owners will let us come in and visit next time we're in town. Her optimism makes me smile.

I do have some pictures from this past week (when my camera wasn't on the fritz!), and I'll have to get those posted. We'll keep everyone posted on the upcoming weeks and visits to clinic. We do have the Relay for Life coming up in the next month on May 1st (http://main.acsevents.org/goto/teamprincesstaylor) ,and the timing will fall about a week after Taylor's biopsy...so many things going on at once, but what an amazing event! Consider joining our team....just click on the link above for Team Princess Taylor. We'd love to have you there!!!

Love to all! Love, Rob, Kim, Taylor, and Alex

April 25, 2009

Shands called yesterday and said Taylor's biopsy from this past Tuesday was clear of Leukemia or anything that they would consider 'abnormal!' The doctor did say that they saw something they call "early recovery cells," which he explained were common and were cells that had been impacted by chemo. I asked him if that is what the pathologist may have seen last time, and he said that most likely it was and that those cells had been categorized as abnormal- but that in actuality- these cells were nothing to worry about.

So- with that news, we are thrilled!

We got the phone call right before I headed out to spend some time with Taylor at her school's field day. She had a great time at field day, and in a weird way- as I watched her do the various relay races, tug of war, etc....I felt (for the first time in a long time) that everything might actually be getting back to normal.

It was a great day to get the news, as we were having our Team Princess Taylor team drop-in last night- and it was great to share the news! I will admit that we had been a bit anxious all week while we waited for a follow-up call. When Taylor was at clinic on Monday, her counts looked great (ANC over 3000, with all of her blood counts continuing to climb as expected). She had the follow-up biopsy on Tuesday morning, and the doctors said that they would rush the results, and that there was a chance we'd have the results on Tuesday. When we still didn't have word on Thursday, we didn't know what to think. On Friday morning I just said a quick prayer and asked for any news- good or bad- just so we would know what to do next....and then the phone call came within a couple of hours....You would think that I would know by now that "letting go" of the situation and turning it over to God is when things happen...guess I just needed that reminder :)

Taylor is continuing to take her weekend antibiotics, which help to ward off infection as her counts / immunity build back up....but that's it for medicine! We'll continue monthly visits to Shands, so she'll head back at the end of May for a check-up and lab work....and I'm assuming they will schedule the surgery to remove her port over the next couple of months. So- things continue to move along here at the Koegel household!

So now we will look ahead to this week's Relay for Life and Team Princess Taylor getting together for the walk! (http:// main.acsevents.org/goto/teamprincesstaylor)

There is still time to sign up for the event- so consider joining us at the event this Friday night!

Love to all, and thank you for continuing to follow this journey...Love, Rob, Kim, Taylor, and Alex

May 4, 2009

The Relay for Life was this past Friday night- what a great event! I was so proud to be a part of Team Princess Taylor- what an amazing group of folks!!! We had coverage all night- at least one person on the track throughout the event....even into those wee hours of the morning....I'm still recovering a bit, as it has taken me a couple of days to stay awake long enough to write this update....

I can't say enough thank yous to the team and to everyone who turned out to show their support. The theme this year was "Every day is a Holiday," and Taylor had picked Hallow- een as our tent's theme. We took the theme and turned it into "Princess Taylor's Pumpkin Patch" and had some great decorations, including a HUGE inflatable pumpkin that lit up. (Thank you Faith Presbyterian for loaning us these great decorations- The light up pumpkin looked great as it got dark outside!) Miss Sarah Cooksey coordinated some great pumpkin patch t-shirts (they were adorable!!!) All of the dec- orations and themes aside, the event itself was simply amaz- ing- over 50 teams, over $50K raised, and amazing fellow- ship. Team Carson was at the campsite next to us, and it was great to see both of the kids doing so well. Carson will wrap up treatment within the next year, and as I watched Taylor and Carson run around- I couldn't help but to think about those early days of being at Shands when both kids were going through those initial days of Induction- and just felt so blessed to see them where they are today.

I was just so appreciative of our amazing team- to wake up at 3 a.m., step outside of the tent and see Scott and Karen still making their laps....to see Grandpa finish his 15+miles he committed to....to have Angie, Anoush, and others com- pleting miles after miles at odd hours of the night, for Rob and Craig who set the campsite up....for Jason who showed up with doughnuts at 4:30 a.m. and to break down the camp- site (and to walk a few more laps too!)- thank you SO much. To everyone who brought out their kids, walked those laps, and supported this event- thank you! And to those that supported us "behind the scenes"- Miss Kathryn with her yummy ribbon chocolates, Grandma and Aunt Debbie for watching the kids late Friday night- all of it helped so much!

After the Relay wrapped up, we continued to have a busy (but fun!) weekend...the kids had 2 birthday parties, Daddy had softball games...lots to do! But all continues to go well, and we count our blessings every day. Taylor will head back to Shands in a couple of weeks for her labs and check-up, and we'll just take each visit one at a time. I'm assuming that this next visit will also include discussion of scheduling the surgery to remove her port....it is interesting because Taylor has asked a lot of questions about this lately- specifically whether she has to have her "buddy" out before her dance recital. She told me that she doesn't want to have it out before her dance recital because she is afraid that she would have to miss the recital. I assured her that we would schedule around that. She really is not in a rush to have her port taken out- the doctors have mentioned this to us in the past...that kids become pretty attached to their "buddy," and that some get sad about having to have it taken out. I guess I can understand why- it has been her friend for the past couple of years- keeping her away from "needle pokes" and providing a standard way for getting medicine and drawing blood for labs....but I'm sure that when it is time for all of this to happen, she will approach it with the same courage with which she has approached the rest of this journey....she is such a trooper.

Well, we'll keep everyone posted on her upcoming trip to Shands and any other happenings- and thank you again for keeping up with her journey.

Love, Rob, Kim, Taylor, and Alex

May 7, 2009

Over the past 2 1/2 years, there have been Caring bridge sites that I check in on from time to time- some of these children have completed treatment....some are still in treatment, some have earned their angel wings....but all have had to experience this cancer journey as a child. When I logged on this morning, it was apparent that there has been a good bit of discussion (on various sites) about political undertones / initiatives regarding childhood cancer. I will admit that to date, my main focus has been getting Taylor through treatment. While I did some minimal reading about current

legislation, stats, etc.- none of it changed the current focus-getting Taylor healthy. I will make more of an effort now to understand legislation that impacts ongoing cancer research, petitions that are out there, etc.....but I found the following excerpt on various sites this morning, and it really struck me. I won't take credit for crafting this following message, but it was an interesting read, and just makes you think.....(Thank you Sandy and Lorie for posting). And while the skeptic in me would love to validate every number prior to posting- my gut tells me that this info probably isn't far off. Just give it a

read with an open mind and don't take offense to other political references in there- the important stats to me were things like the lack of pediatric cancer drugs available right now:

"The following contrasts H1N1 to the childhood cancer crisis:

The Swine Flu: A Crisis? You Decide!!!

It's all over the news. The Swine Flu has entered the U.S., and everyone is responding quickly. Here is what has happened already:

--Over 100 schools have closed.

--President Obama called on all schools with possible swine flu cases to "strongly consider temporarily closing."

--Congress approved $1.5 billion in emergency funds.

--Education Secretary Arne Duncan said that everyone involved in schools needs to "pitch in and do our part to prevent the spread of this flu virus."

--The Department of Education and the CDC have held conferences to give updates and advice for handling the crisis.

--WHO Director-General Margaret Chan has raised the alert level to phase 5.

--Shipments of the drug Tamiflu from the federal stockpile, enough to treat 11 million patients, have been distributed to several states.

--Dr. Jesse Goodman, of the Food and Drug Administration's swine flu work said, "We're working together at 100 miles an hour."

--Congress has asked Homeland to consider closing the Mexican border.

Here are the numbers: There have been 84 documented cases in the U.S. There has been one death, a two-year-old boy with underlying health issues.

Updates on the Swine Flu epidemic are all over the papers, T.V., Internet, and radio. You can't avoid it.

This is a crisis and deserves a fast response. Sick children, and the death of even one child, is a great loss. But I am a little confused. I would like to point out some comparisons.

1) Since the outbreak in the U.S., there have been 84 cases of swine flu, and one death.

Compare that to the fact that 12,600 families are told their child has cancer each year. That is 35 families every single day of the year.

2) The media tells us that the 84 cases and one death from the swine flu is a "crisis" and "epidemic". But do a google search on childhood cancer, and you will find the media consistently touts childhood cancer, with 40,000 current cases and 2,500 annual deaths, as "very rare".

3) To protect yourself against the swine flu, you should wash hands, not touch your nose, and cover your mouth. You can

even wear gloves and a mask. But there is no protection against childhood cancers. In fact, the cause of most childhood cancers is still unknown.

4) The swine flu produces severe flu symptoms. The effects of cancer are beyond description. So just consider this: Cancer is part of the body, so the treatment is a process of poisoning the child to the brink of death, then pulling back hoping they stabilize, then hitting them again. Over and over and over. Maybe a year, maybe 7 years. The resulting organ failures often cause more complications and deaths than the cancer itself. And then you wait and pray that it all worked. "Remission" only means they think they got it. "Relapse" means they were wrong.

5) The government has opened up its stockpile of flu drugs to fight the crisis. But there is no stockpile of cancer drugs. In fact, it has been 30 years since a new pediatric cancer drug has been developed. A 5-year study by the National Institute of Health concluded that new drugs for pediatric and adolescent cancers are not being developed because the profit margins are too slim. Therefore, mega-doses of adult chemotherapy are administered to children.

6) Congress has approved $1.5 billion in ADDITIONAL funding to fight the swine flu. With 84 infected people, that is $18 million per person. Childhood cancer received a TOTAL of $30 million over a 5-year period. That works out to $750 for each child currently fighting cancer.

So, does any of this scare you more than the swine flu? It should. The emergency response to the swine flu has been great. But where is the emergency plan for childhood cancer? And where is the media attention? There is none.

Some might say these are not fair comparisons. Well, in one way they would be correct. The $1.5 billion for the flu has been paid. The $30 million for childhood cancer was approved by the federal government as the Carolyn Walker Pryce Childhood Cancer Act, but has never been funded.

Other issues of greater crisis keep taking priority, such as $120 million to distribute free condoms in 3rd world countries (Yes, really. It's in the stimulus package).

Some might still say my comparisons are still unfair, that I am not comparing apples to apples. But, just for the record, the U.S. apple growers got $170 million in the stimulus package.

Honestly, I am not criticizing the response to the Swine Flu. It is an appropriate response. I just do not understand why our children with cancer deserve less.

Please remember:
1 in 300 children will be diagnosed with cancer before the age of 20.
12,600 children are diagnosed each year.
3,000 will die of cancer each year.
Cancer is the #1 disease killer of children ages 1-19.
The cause of most childhood cancers is still unknown.
Only 3% of cancer research money goes toward childhood cancers.
There are currently 30,000-40,000 children fighting cancer in the U.S.
The number of children diagnosed with cancer has increased every year for the past 25 years.

Teenagers and young adults (ages 15-22) are the only age group that have flat or declining survival rates from cancer.

In the past 35 years ONLY ONE new cancer drug has been approved for pediatric use.

Since children can handle much more chemo than adults, most treatments are little more than mega doses of adult cancer chemotherapy treatments. The result of these high doses of chemo on children is a higher rate of secondary cancers.

For reasons not fully known, teenagers experience the highest rate of secondary cancers as a result of the high dose chemotherapy treatments.

Teenagers have the highest cancer fatality rate of any age group under 80. Their cancers tend to be much more rare, therefore lacking established treatments. Their cancers also tend to be far more advanced when diagnosed.

A 5-year study at Children's Hospital Pittsburgh of UPMC recently concluded that teenage cancer survivorship is lower due in part to a lack of access to clinical trials. They concluded: "Patients who are enrolled in clinical trials offering the most advanced cancer treatments do better than patients who receive conventional treatment. Adolescents and young adults with cancer are less likely than younger children to be enrolled in clinical trials."

This entry was copied off of the PAC2 Website http://cure-childhoodcancer.ning.com/"

May 21, 2009

Let me start by sending thanks to Miss Kaitlyn for her compassion (and determination) with her recent donation to Locks Of Love (a non-profit organization that helps in providing wigs / hair prosthetics for children experiencing long term hair loss....). Kaitlyn began growing out her hair in 2007 when Taylor was diagnosed with Leukemia- and she just had her big hair cut this week!!! What an amazing little girl...I'll admit that when I launched this picture from her Mommy's email, I was pretty choked up....

So- another big trip to Shands today. Taylor and Rob left early this morning for her monthly check-up. It's hard to explain, because for so long we wished for the chemo to be done- but with the medicine complete, there is just a good bit of anxiety as we wait for her counts. My heart tells me to accept each day as it comes- but my head was counting down the days until her trip to Gainesville so that we could see the lab results and know that everything is okay. Thankfully, all of her blood counts came back in normal ranges (with the exception of her white blood cell count)- but her doctors told Rob that it may take a full 6 months for those to rebound. Her doctors don't seem to be concerned, but Rob and I do have some questions about her ANC, as it was ~1800...which was lower than her last visit- but again, her doctors don't seem to be concerned. I'll probably call them tomorrow just to understand if there is an assumed range of fluctuation....Rob asked the doctor today when the "nauseous feeling stops..."- that tight feeling in the pit of your stomach when Taylor takes an extra nap....or wakes up looking slightly pale....or that maybe we're just reading more into a situation than we should be....The doctor said that it just takes time. I'm sure it does.

I was so proud of both of the girls tonight- as they had their dress rehearsal for their dance recital this coming weekend. They both did amazing- especially little Alex who was okay with me going to sit in the audience while she was backstage all by herself! (She is a big kid now- or so she tells us...) They both were beaming as they did their routines, and I was just so happy for both of them. Taylor also had her first sleepover with a friend from school this past weekend- and she had a blast. The girls had been planning it for at least the past 2 months! With everything they had on their agenda...we may need to schedule a few more sleepovers this summer to get through their list of planned activities :)

I guess what I try to do is just take all of these normal things going on and treasure them. Whether it is a dance recital or an end of year party for school- no event feels small anymore. I think one of the things that Rob and I have been treasuring a lot is Taylor's newfound love of reading to us. Now that the whole reading thing has clicked for her- she wants to read and read and read every night...falling asleep with books in bed....it's adorable. Even with all of her reading though, she still likes Mommy or Daddy to read at least one book per night. Last night I was reading her one of my favorite kid books called "Hooray for You"- and there is a passage that I love to read to her (although it chokes me up from time to time)...it reads as follows:

"On the day you were born, the world grew by one; Life with big purpose and much to be done.
Look in the mirror. Love who you see.
Stand tall. Smile big. Shout Hooray for Me!"

I just look at her and see such a strong little girl who can take on anything....I hope she sees the same thing too...

Well, I need to sign off for now- lots to do yet tonight...but wanted to send love to everyone and we will keep you posted on Taylor's progress.

Love, Rob, Kim, Taylor, and Alex

June 6, 2009

Just wanted to check in and let everyone know that things continue to go well here in the Koegel household. Taylor and Alex continue to amaze me with their energy....the end of the school year has just been such a busy time! The girls had their big dance recital the Saturday of Memorial Day weekend, and they were just adorable! I posted some pictures, and was just smiling as I went through them again tonight. The girls just looked so beautiful. Alex was not pleased about taking pictures, but we did manage to snap a few! Following Memorial Day weekend, it was the last week of school (complete with all sorts of fun activities), and then we have now rolled into summer....and Taylor's first year of summer camp and all that it includes (lots of daily, fun activities)....and the girls are heading into Week 2 of swim lessons....Whew- we've been busy!

But busy is so good....so normal. It is very nice. I was talking with friends last night trying to explain how amazing it is for Taylor to be done with her medicine. Yes, there continues to be Septra (an antibiotic Taylor takes while her immune system builds back up), but there is no more chemo. What continues to amaze me is how quickly our family has been willing to put that part of it behind us. There has just been no need to dwell- it's not like it was a fun time, and I remember hating seeing the impacts it was having on her body...some she continues to recover from. But- regardless, we have been more than happy to move on with life with no chemotherapy. I received a phone call today from the mom of a little boy here in Tallahassee who was recently diagnosed with the same type of Leukemia. Thankfully, he has now entered 'Consolidation' (the phase following Induction for Leukemia, ALL treatment). She was worried because his appetite is up and down- so big on the steroids, not as big now- his tastes have changed- how should she get him to eat more, etc....I took a deep breath as she explained what was going on, knowing that she and her family still have such a long road ahead, but I was happy to be able to talk to her and share our experiences with her. Support networks are so important for families as they navigate this journey, and if we haven't told all of you today, thank you again for being that network for us.

We will keep everyone posted on Taylor's upcoming Shands visit (scheduled for later this month). Rob and I continue to learn about what types of blood count fluctuations are considered acceptable, and just take each visit one day at a time. In our hearts, we just continue to appreciate each day that God gives us together as a family. Life is good...

Before I sign off, I did want to thank Jennifer Brucker (Miss Kathryn's sister) who is taking on the challenge of Team in Training!

http://pages.teamintraining.org/sc/nikesf09/jbrucker

Best of luck to her and her team mates as they prepare for their run, and continue to support fundraising for Leukemia research.

Love to all, and we'll post more soon. Love, Rob, Kim, Taylor, and Alex

June 18, 2009

Taylor and Rob headed down to Shands for Taylor's monthly check-up today. All went well, with an ANC of 2600! One of the most interesting things to Rob was the fact that her lab values are in normal ranges (with the exception of her white blood cell count- which the doctors are okay with- they still expect that at this point). Having said that though, her white blood cell count was at 4.5! Again, I know that number may not mean a lot without context, but that value is 4 times what it was at some points during treatment! It is just an amazing feeling to see her continue to progress through this journey, and tackle it all regardless of the toll it has taken. The doctors explained that we will meet with a pediatric surgeon next month to discuss removing her port (a.k.a, her "buddy"). To date, Taylor hasn't been thrilled at the fact that the doctors want her buddy back. She is fine with it staying put. (As a matter of fact, it is a nice option for ongoing blood draws too). I guess I can understand why she has no intent of letting them take her buddy...in the beginning, there is a lot of focus on helping the kids understand how the port will be "a friend" to them...help them avoid needle pokes, etc. It is part of this whole journey to her...but- it is the next logical step in moving past this whole ordeal- so we will help her get past this too.

This morning was a bit of a battle to get her in the car to Gainesville. She was just so mad at Rob and me- "How dare we make her late for summer camp!!!" She couldn't believe that we would schedule clinic for a day she had camp- especially a day they were going swimming! "Take me to clinic on Saturday Mommy- not today!!!" We were "the meanest parents ever." After a lot of patient discussions, (and finally Rob giving an ultimatum of having to miss 2 days of summer camp if she didn't get in the car soon)- they were on their way. I guess the flip side is that she is truly enjoying summer camp- so that makes us happy too.

So- we'll keep everyone posted on Miss Taylor and upcoming appointments. We just continue to take one day at a time and thank God for all of the blessings and continued perspective he has given us through this journey.

Love to all, and we will post more soon.

Love, Rob, Kim, Taylor, and Alex

July 25, 2009

It has been a busy summer- with lots to update about. Most importantly, Taylor and Rob went to Shands this past Thursday for Taylor's monthly check-up. The doctors were happy with her counts (ANC of 1500), and said she had a growth spurt too! Her white blood cell count continues to hover around 4, which at first was something Rob and I questioned, but her doctors seem okay with it. They feel confident that her immunity will continue to rebuild now that she is done with chemo, and that it will climb. They also talked to us about starting daily vitamins (like Flintstones or something). Rob and I laughed after I bought them because she has no idea who the Flintstones are...

So, we continue to give her Septra weekly (the antibiotic she'll take for a period of time while immunity rebuilds), and just continue to be thankful for her progress. It's just a weird cycle. We get through the month doing "normal" things now, not worrying about timing at night for medicine, etc.- but that 1 day each month is nauseating. The 45 minutes it takes between a blood draw and the results coming back seem more like 45 hours, and then you just try to dismiss any fears and remember that it is out of your hands....And I give a lot of credit to Rob- because he continues to handle the bulk of the visits over the past year...and while I may be thinking about it from afar...he is there with the reality of it all staring him in the face. I thank God for him all of the time.

During their visit, Rob also talked with the pediatric surgeon about timing for taking out Taylor's port. She reiterated that there is not a rush to take it out, and maybe we look ahead to Christmas break. It should be outpatient surgery, and sounds pretty standard...so for now, we may just leave well enough alone.

So, now onto one of the highlights of summer....we took a family trip to Aruba. This was a trip that we had originally planned in 2007, but for obvious reasons, we put the trip on hold...but it was a trip we eventually wanted to do. Taylor had been there once before (when she was just shy of 2 years old, and I was pregnant with Alex). So, it was exciting to be able to go back- and just a big trip for everyone- Alex's first trip on a plane and using a passport, Taylor's first-time snorkeling, the girls' first time on a big sailboat...and lots of swimming for everyone! Uncle Joel and Aunt Peg (from North Carolina) made the trip down too! It was an amazing trip, and we were there over Taylor's 6th birthday too which was nice. I've posted several pictures from the trip, and the one resounding theme from the trip was that no one wanted to come back home! One thing I really loved about being there was that our cell phones didn't work- In fact, most people you saw did not have one....so there was not a ton of people talking on phones, texting all the time- or just rushing around in general. Everything just seems to move on island time there- I could get used to that! So, we are back home now and tried to get back in the swing of things this week. Taylor is back at summer camp, Alex is at school, and Rob and I are back at work. Our house is getting an unexpected mini-renovation, as we had some plumbing issues that have now resulted in replumbing the house...which leads to a couple of other projects...dry wall, painting, etc...but in the scheme of things, I'll take that any day.

So, all in all, life is good. The kids are enjoying summer, and all reports from Shands continue to show progress. School starts next month- and it is hard to believe that Taylor will be starting 1st grade. It is a miracle in itself, and reminds me every day that God's grace is what continues to make all of this possible.

Love to everyone, and we'll update more soon!

Love, Rob, Kim, Taylor, and Alex

August 13, 2009

I'm not quite sure how to start this journal entry- so I will simply just ask for your prayers. It is a long story, but the end result is that we are awaiting a bone marrow biopsy in the morning to understand if Taylor's Leukemia has relapsed.

It all started when we were driving South today- in fact, on the way to funeral services for my grandfather- an amazing man who passed away last Saturday. With all that is going on, I know that Taylor has yet another angel watching over her, and I know that Grandpa understands why Rob and I are in Gainesville tonight instead of being able to attend services in his honor.

It was today that Taylor was to have her monthly visit to Shands as well- and we figured we could stop on the way down to South Florida, get counts checked, and be on our way. Instead, Dr. Slayton asked if he could talk to Rob and I alone- specifically about some concerning drops in Taylor's platelet and white blood cell counts. Our hearts just dropped- knowing that we were about to hear the words that we had so hoped we would not have to. Dr. Slayton believes that there is a chance that Taylor's Leukemia is relapsing, and he scheduled a bone marrow biopsy for first thing tomorrow morning to confirm. We should have results tomorrow, and then know what the next steps are. I'm sure I don't have to explain how hard this is to even comprehend- we have just wanted to close this chapter for Taylor and move on, but we will see tomorrow if God has yet a bigger plan for this that we don't yet understand.

We spent today doing some swimming, going to the movies, eating popcorn until we nearly exploded, and just trying to distract ourselves from the painful "waiting" that comes with yet another procedure.

Taylor is older now, and she is aware of what is going on. When we left clinic today, she looked me square in the eyes and asked me "Mommy, do people with cancer sometimes die?" It took everything I had in me to look her back in the eyes and be honest, but I promised her I would never lie to her. Before I could even say anything though- (I guess she could tell just from my delay)- she responded with "That means Yes...." I took a deep breath and just explained that "Yes sweetheart, sometimes they do, but sometimes they don't." And then- it was off to find a hotel with a swimming pool. If by chance she is going to be cooped up in a hospital in the coming weeks- there was no way we weren't going to make the most of today.

I am trying my best to keep it all together- and just asking God for the strength to hear whatever news we get tomorrow. While I know what we selfishly want the news to be, we also have to be prepared for the tough answer of a relapse and next steps....testing for bone marrow donors, possible redo of chemo for the next 27 months...not exactly sure where this will head. But I do know that we have a strong support network and that Rob and I have each other- and that we will do everything we can to get through this. I will admit that I have already had thoughts today about the fact that school is starting in just a little over a week....that she is going into 1st grade- and that this just isn't fair....but I really am trying to remind myself to take it one step at a time, and just try to get through today.

We will post as soon as we know the outcome of the biopsy. If I had to ask for specific prayers- it would be for strength- strength for Taylor's body and strength for all of us as we brace for an update tomorrow.

Love to all- and thank you again for your support of us in this journey.

Love, Rob, Kim, Taylor, and Alex

August 13, 2009

I'm not quite sure how to start this journal entry- so I will simply just ask for your prayers. It is a long story, but the end result is that we are awaiting a bone marrow biopsy in the morning to understand if Taylor's Leukemia has relapsed.

It all started when we were driving South today- in fact, on the way to funeral services for my grandfather- an amazing man who passed away last Saturday. With all that is going on, I know that Taylor has yet another angel watching over her, and I know that Grandpa understands why Rob and I are in Gainesville tonight instead of being able to attend services in his honor.

It was today that Taylor was to have her monthly visit to Shands as well- and we figured we could stop on the way down to South Florida, get counts checked, and be on our way. Instead, Dr. Slayton asked if he could talk to Rob and I alone- specifically about some concerning drops in Taylor's platelet and white blood cell counts. Our hearts just dropped- knowing that we were about to hear the words that we had so hoped we would not have to. Dr. Slayton believes that there is a chance that Taylor's Leukemia is relapsing, and he scheduled a bone marrow biopsy for first thing tomorrow morning to confirm. We should have results tomorrow, and then know what the next steps are. I'm sure I don't have to explain how hard this is to even comprehend- we have just wanted to close this chapter for Taylor and move on, but we will see tomorrow if God has yet a bigger plan for this that we don't yet understand.

We spent today doing some swimming, going to the movies, eating popcorn until we nearly exploded, and just trying to distract ourselves from the painful "waiting" that comes with yet another procedure.

Taylor is older now, and she is aware of what is going on.

When we left clinic today, she looked me square in the eyes and asked me "Mommy, do people with cancer sometimes die?" It took everything I had in me to look her back in the eyes and be honest, but I promised her I would never lie to her. Before I could even say anything though- (I guess she could tell just from my delay)- she responded with "That means Yes...." I took a deep breath and just explained that "Yes sweetheart, sometimes they do, but sometimes they don't." And then- it was off to find a hotel with a swimming pool. If by chance she is going to be cooped up in a hospital in the coming weeks- there was no way we weren't going to make the most of today.

I am trying my best to keep it all together- and just asking God for the strength to hear whatever news we get tomorrow. While I know what we selfishly want the news to be, we also have to be prepared for the tough answer of a relapse and next steps....testing for bone marrow donors, possible redo of chemo for the next 27 months...not exactly sure where this will head. But I do know that we have a strong support network and that Rob and I have each other- and that we will do everything we can to get through this. I will admit that I have already had thoughts today about the fact that school is starting in just a little over a week....that she is going into 1st grade- and that this just isn't fair....but I really am trying to remind myself to take it one step at a time, and just try to get through today.

We will post as soon as we know the outcome of the biopsy. If I had to ask for specific prayers- it would be for strength- strength for Taylor's body and strength for all of us as we brace for an update tomorrow. Love to all- and thank you again for your support of us in this journey.

Love, Rob, Kim, Taylor, and Alex

August 14, 2009

Let us start by saying "Thank You" to everyone. Your posts, calls, texts, and support have meant so much, and continue to lift our spirits.

I wish I had more to tell you- but we just don't know the answer yet....but I did want to post something, as I know the silence can be scary....

Taylor had her biopsy early this morning, and we are now just waiting on a call from Shands with a confirmed Pathology report on whether or not there is a relapse.

The silence today was killing us though- and so finally, late this afternoon, I called Shands. Dr. Slayton returned our call, and he told us that he didn't want to give us false hope- but that the slide he was reviewing didn't appear to have Leukemia cells. He was clear though that we had to wait for a Pathology report to have a better sense of whether there is a relapse or not....but this was a glimmer of hope that we did not have yesterday- and that was something, and has given us more hope as we continue to wait for that call.

It was a strange morning though- because when we left the surgery center, we literally did not know where we were driving to....They had not yet admitted her (because the doctors didn't know if she had relapsed), but we were waiting on the results- so do you stay? And while one of her doctors said we would know today- another one told us this morning it could be 48 hours- so do you go? We did know that Taylor missed Alex miserably, so we just started driving in that general direction- and ended up driving to Orlando to meet up with Grandma, Grandpa, and Alex.

As we drove, Rob and I agreed that while we waited for that call- we were going to pack in as much fun for her as we possibly could (and as much as she felt comfortable doing). We had originally thought about going to Disney in October and going to a place called the "Bibbity Bobbity Boutique" (i.e.., a princess boutique where the girls get to dress up like a princess, get their hair done, etc.)- but as we drove, and with so many uncertainties about where Taylor would even be in October with regard to treatment- we decided to accelerate things a bit. I know it sounds harsh, but if treatment was to start again, Taylor would lose her hair again as well, and so we wanted to do the appointments sooner than later. So, by some miracle- we were able to get appointments for both girls today- and through some teary eyes, we watched two little girls have a blast today. Taylor dressed up like Belle, and Alex dressed up like a "Bride" (she told us that she was Princess Aurora). They were precious, and it somehow seemed to ease some of the anxiety that Taylor has been feeling the past 2 days.

It's just hard- we can't even comprehend what is going on in her mind, but we know she is scared. She told us this morning that she doesn't want to die....and we told her that we will do everything in our power to fight these cancer germs. Then she asked me "But what if I do?" And I told her "Then you will be in the most amazing place you can be...." And she said "I know."

It's just a roller coaster ride, and I thank all of you again for your support through this.

If we know something tonight, I'll post more...we are just waiting on that call, and are just so hopeful that it will not show a relapse. If that is the case, we will thank God for yet another opportunity to spend more time together as a family, and then we'll just take it one step at a time.

Love to all, and thank you so much. Love, Rob, Kim, Taylor, and Alex

August 15, 2009

Thank you again to everyone for your calls and messages of support. We reached out to Shands again today to check and see if there was a status update on the Pathology report. We are still waiting to hear, but promise to post as soon as we have an update.

There are lots of things that bring us strength and hope- including the fact that Taylor's energy seems unlimited...in fact, that is another reason all of this took us by complete surprise on Thursday when the doctors appeared so concerned with her counts.

The past few days are really just a blur- and I can't necessarily explain all of our emotions. I know it may seem crazy that we ended up at a Disney princess boutique yesterday, and I hope it did not appear that we were being irresponsible....it's just that your heart breaks for her if this truly is a relapse- and in all honesty, I would have rented the space shuttle yesterday if she had told me she wanted to travel to the moon....it's just where your head is at this point- I don't want her to miss out on anything. Most importantly though, it is just important to us right now to keep her distracted from all of this anxiety. I had just never seen her doctors so worried about a set of labs to date....and there had been times when her counts had dipped before....and they are not quick to do a bone marrow biopsy...When there were concerns in the past, and we asked "Is it possible to do a bone marrow biopsy?" The doctors said "No- we would only do that if the blood work gave us true concern that there was a relapse...." That may give everyone some more context as to why we have been so distraught over the past few days. But no matter how unsettled Rob and I are feeling, I think we realized that sitting in a hotel crying for 2 days wasn't helping the situation either...we needed to be out living life with Taylor and Alex.

I just pray that all of this is a big mistake- but I also remember that we are not the first to walk this path. There are other families out there that have had to deal with this news...or the roller coaster of up and down emotions of waiting for results. I guess what I'm trying to say is that I feel like we are in a much better place today than we were on Thursday- regardless of the outcome. While I know what we want the outcome to be, I think we've gotten a lot of the emotional outbursts out of the way and are ready to face whatever comes.

So- I am hoping to post an update soon- although it still could be another day while Pathology continues to run the full spectrum of tests to figure out what the heck is going on.

Thank you, thank you, and thank you again for your prayers. Love, Rob, Kim, Taylor, and Alex

August 17, 2009

Shands called this afternoon with some frustrating news- somehow the lab misplaced Taylor's biopsy sample from Friday. I was just in disbelief- how could this happen?

As my mind was starting to race about having to take Taylor for yet another biopsy, the person on the phone explained that Dr. Slayton had taken an extra sample on Friday for his own review and that he was able to ship that sample over to the lab this afternoon...and that we should have a result in the morning.

Yes, we are extremely frustrated, and I'll take time to be angry later- but no matter how angry I am right now- no amount of yelling or kicking something is going to get the results any faster. I just feel sick about it though...

I will pass along something that was supportive yesterday though...a book I've mentioned in previous entries- a daily devotional called "Streams in the Desert." It had been awhile since I had reached for that book, but last night I really needed to read something to give me just a little bit of reassurance- and there it was when I opened the page...the August 16th posting was about "Waiting." There was a particular part that stood out to me, and I read the whole entry to Rob...it said "But God has a purpose in all of his holdups. The steps of a good man are ordered by the Lord."(Psalm 37:23)

It is amazing how I picked up that book at just the right time yesterday. And I'm not sure what the purpose of this holdup is...or the confusion with the lab sample- but I am doing my best to not be frustrated while we do wait.

Hopefully I will be able to post some results soon. Love to

all...Love, Rob, Kim, Taylor, and Alex

August 18, 2009

The marrow is clear!!! Dr. Slayton just called!!!

I can't even explain how Rob and I are feeling right now- we have just been sick about this, and to get this news- the tears of thanks just started flowing.

All of that said, we will have follow-up checks on her counts in the next couple of weeks to continue monitoring her progress- but whatever caused the drop in her counts does not appear to be a Leukemia relapse.

Thank you, thank you, thank you for your prayers and support. It all means so much and has carried us through this difficult time over the past 6 days.

Love to all, and I will post more soon- I just want to get this posted ASAP!

Love, Rob, Kim, Taylor, and Alex

August 29, 2009

The girls had a great first week of school! Taylor started first grade and Alex started her new class at preschool!

We celebrated the end of a "good first week" with a fort and movie night last night and some popcorn... Taylor still gets excited about getting to have a snack at night time and not having to worry about 6-MP or Methotrexate. It truly is some of the smallest things in life that can be the most precious...Rob and I will be talking with Shands on Monday about Taylor's next appointment there (i.e., whether we just get her counts checked here or whether they will see her in person there). After everything that happened a couple weeks ago with the scare with her counts, my gut says we'll be headed to Shands for a visit- but that's okay. The biopsy was the last "check" of her counts, etc.....so we are hopeful that her white blood cell count and her platelets are continuing to come back up. It's hard to explain how it is something constantly on your mind- yet you try to not think about it...

because there's not really a thing you can do about it....and it's not like we're in control of any of this anyway! We just remain thankful for a clear biopsy, a happy child, and things like getting to start school this year. There are sadly too many children that did not get to do that this year. When I see how much Taylor enjoys school and her after school program, I remember to thank God for the fact that she was okay and able to head back to school with her friends.

So- with that, we are just looking ahead to the Fall and all that it brings- school activities, dance class, golf camp for Taylor, Football games, the holidays...so much to enjoy! We will keep everyone posted on news from Shands next week, and wanted to thank you again for the outpouring of support you've continued to show our family. Leukemia has been a long journey- one that I could not have envisioned when all of this started....but thank you again for following Taylor.

Love, Rob, Kim, Taylor, and Alex

August 29, 2009

The girls had a great first week of school! Taylor started first grade and Alex started her new class at preschool!

We celebrated the end of a "good first week" with a fort and movie night last night and some popcorn... Taylor still gets excited about getting to have a snack at night time and not having to worry about 6-MP or Methotrexate. It truly is some of the smallest things in life that can be the most precious...

Rob and I will be talking with Shands on Monday about Taylor's next appointment there (i.e., whether we just get her counts checked here or whether they will see her in person there). After everything that happened a couple weeks ago with the scare with her counts, my gut says we'll be headed to Shands for a visit- but that's okay. The biopsy was the last "check" of her counts, etc.....so we are hopeful that her white blood cell count and her platelets are continuing to come back up. It's hard to explain how it is something constantly on your mind- yet you try to not think about it...because there's not really a thing you can do about it....and it's not like we're in control of any of this anyway! We just remain thankful for a clear biopsy, a happy child, and things like getting to start school this year. There are sadly too many children that did not get to do that this year. When I see how much Taylor enjoys school and her after school program, I remember to thank God for the fact that she was okay and able to head back to school with her friends.

So- with that, we are just looking ahead to the Fall and all that it brings- school activities, dance class, golf camp for Taylor, Football games, the holidays...so much to enjoy! We will keep everyone posted on news from Shands next week, and wanted to thank you again for the outpouring of support you've continued to show our family. Leukemia has been a long journey- one that I could not have envisioned when all of this started....but thank you again for following Taylor.

Love, Rob, Kim, Taylor, and Alex

September 2, 2009

Taylor and Daddy headed over to KidsKorner bright and early on Tuesday morning so that she could get her labs done before heading off to school....

Rob got a call from KidsKorner pretty quickly saying that all of Taylor's labs were in normal range! Her white blood cells were back up to 4, and her platelets were over 180. When Rob called me, I just took such a big sigh of relief and just said a quick prayer of thanks. It was just such comforting news to see her white blood cell count and platelets heading back in the right direction, and it helped reinforce the outcome of the biopsy a couple of weeks ago. Shands called within a couple of hours and they were happy with the counts as well...in fact, they feel comfortable enough for Taylor to just have counts checked here in September again...and not head back to Shands until October. That is a big step!

So, while we know the journey will continue and there will always be bouts of worry- it was nice to have comforting news yesterday.

We'll keep you posted on her progress, and thank you again for all of your kind words, prayers and support for our family. Love, Rob, Kim, Taylor, and Alex

September 22, 2009

As I write this tonight, Taylor and Alex have yet another angel in heaven watching over them. Rob called just a short time ago to let us know that Gammy (Rob's mom) has passed away. While my heart feels heavy right now, we are grateful that it was possible to have Hospice care for Gammy and allow her the peace of being home with Rob and his sisters for her last couple of days here on Earth.

Telling the girls was tough- but truly, children have such an amazing way of taking some of life's toughest moments and bringing such a purity to them that only a child can....

The 3 of us prayed together tonight at bedtime, and asked God to take care of Gammy. Alex asked that "God take care of Gammy, Grandpa Herbie and Great Grandpa because those are the only people she can think of in heaven right now." And Taylor wanted to tell Gammy "how much she loved her cookies." And then Alex reminded Taylor and me that "we are all going to heaven someday to see Gammy again- so why is everybody crying?" Yes...the purity of a child's view- it is refreshing.

One silver lining to the journey we have had with Taylor over the past few years is the ongoing, open discussion about spirituality. There is a comfort level with heaven, the fact that our loved ones are there, and that God has a plan- even if it doesn't make sense to us now. I know that it doesn't make sense to them that Gammy is no longer here with us, but it gave me comfort to see them understand that she is in a better place.

Along the lines of children....the girls have been on quite a 'Peter Pan' kick the past few days...not sure why this movie was such a hit with them recently, but it was quite timely. I say that because it was through a simple set of song lyrics this weekend (from a children's movie) that I found such a wonderful way to describe mothers...and of course- it made me think of Gammy...

"Well, a mother, a real mother
Is the most wonderful person in the world She's the angel voice that bids you good night.

Kisses your cheek, whispers, 'Sleep tight'

Your Mother and Mine... Your Mother and Mine...

The helping hand that guides you along Whether you're right, whether you're wrong

Your Mother and Mine... Your Mother and Mine...

What makes mothers all that they are? Might as well ask 'What makes a star?' Ask your heart to tell you her worth Your heart will say 'Heaven on Earth'

Another word for divine... Your Mother and Mine..."

So- thank you to everyone who has prayed for Rob and our family over the past week. I ask that you continue to pray for strength and acceptance in the days to come.

Love to all...Love, Rob, Kim, Taylor, and Alex

October 4, 2009

Rob and Taylor headed to KidsKorner bright and early this past Thursday morning so that Taylor could get her labs done before school. When we got the call from TMH (and a subsequent call from Shands) about her labs, we were just amazed and very thankful. Her ANC was over 3700! (with a white blood cell count over 6, hematocrit and hemoglobin of 12 and 35, and platelets at 139...)

While Rob and I were thrilled to see her counts at such a comfortable level- we wanted some sort of reassurance from

Shands about her platelets (after the relapse scare in August). Shands had no concerns, and in fact, they were comfortable enough for Taylor to discontinue her last medicine that she's been taking- her Septra! Septra is an antibiotic that Taylor continued to take 6 months post-treatment. She took it 3 days per week, twice per day to help her body as her immunity built back up- but now we are 6 months post treatment, and her doctors feel okay about how things are going.

When I saw Taylor on Thursday afternoon after school, I told her the news about the Septra. To say she was excited would not do it justice- in fact, she has told nearly everyone she's seen this weekend that she is done with Septra! I will admit that I was very careful about choosing my words about being done with her medicine...I told her "Taylor, your doctors said you are all done with your medicine for right now!" The key words being "right now..." While my heart tells me she is done with medicine forever, my head also reminds me to not make a promise that Rob and I can't deliver on for her..." We pray that she is done forever, but we'll take "right now" for right now.

We'll head down to Shands next week for her a visit, and we'll keep everyone posted on the results of that trip!

This past week has been okay otherwise- the whole family is just trying to get back into the swing of things. The girls ask about their Gammy and heaven often, and I know they miss her dearly. One of the most amazing moments over the past week was during our road trip on the way to Port Saint Lucie...The girls and I were about an hour outside of Port Saint Lucie and we were traveling through a rain storm- and all of a sudden, the most beautiful double rainbow appeared! The colors were brilliant and it spanned across the sky. It was the perfect way to help the girls understand God's promise to us that all will be okay. I was so moved by the rainbow that I had to pull over and take a picture of
it. While the picture does not necessarily do it justice, the

memory of that rainbow will never fade. The girls were sure that it was Gammy and Great Grandpa telling them that everything was going to be fine. I was so thankful that God gave me that opportunity to reinforce the faith of two little girls that day- especially as you are trying to help them understand that there is a reason for all things in life- even the things that make us sad.

Thank you again to everyone for your prayers and kind words over the past couple of weeks (and the past couple of years!) We'll keep you posted on the next round of checkups as this journey continues....Love to all...Love, Rob, Kim, Taylor, and Alex

October 18, 2009

It has been a busy week- and so much to be thankful for....

Most importantly- Taylor had a checkup this past Thursday at Shands, and her counts came back great! Her white blood cells were at 5.9, platelets up to 200, and hematocrit and hemoglobin levels of 13 and 35- When Rob texted me her counts, I was in the middle of a meeting, and my eyes just filled with "happy" tears...A big sigh and a prayer of thanks later, I just thought about how far she has come through all of this. There's not a day that goes by when I don't think about that...but Rob and I agree that the days that she goes to get her counts checked- you just feel sick until you hear the results. Her doctors were happy overall, and mentioned that all should be on track for her "buddy" (i.e., her port) to come out over Christmas break...We'll break that to her as it gets closer- she reminds me that "Nobody is taking her buddy."

Another big event this weekend was Taylor's first race! She participated in her school's "Red Fox Trot" and ran in the 1 mile! I ran with her, and she did amazing! I asked her a couple of times if she was okay or wanted to slow down, and she just said "Let's run faster Mommy!" So- I did my best to keep up with her and we crossed the finish line together. Rob and I were so proud of her!

So- life continues to feel normal again in our household- the girls are keeping busy with school and dance...and Taylor is wrapping up with her golf camp. (Thank you again to the Hanstein family- the clubs are working out great)! She has really enjoyed golf, and is even trying to give her Daddy tips before he heads out to the course....In fact, I went to call him today, and she reminded me it is not good etiquette to call someone and make a loud noise- "What if someone was trying to hit the ball and you messed it up Mommy?" So yes- we continue to have some good laughs too.

Well, love to all- and we will keep you updated on Taylor's progress.

Love, Rob, Kim, Taylor, and Alex

November 21, 2009

Taylor was able to have her check-up locally this month ...so this past Thursday was a welcome change from making a long car trip for her appointment! We had her blood work done here at KidsKorner, and then she was able to see her pediatrician- so while it was still a long afternoon, it was nice to still be here in Tallahassee, and to know that her doctors at Shands feel comfortable with that too. Her labs came back fine, with all of her counts in acceptable ranges. Rob and I still hold our breath while we're waiting for the counts to come back, and we wonder if that will ever change....but regardless, we just remember to be thankful for her continued progress, and that here we are....almost 3 years from when all of this started...

We are thankful that life continues to go along "normally" and that updates to the website are typically monthly after Taylor's appointments....That is a very good thing! Although, as I look back over the past month, there have been a lot of fun things to celebrate....Good check-ups, Halloween, field trips, fun trips to football games, Taylor's first golf tournament (where she placed 2nd and got her first medal!!!)....just a nice, busy, normal month. A little note about that golf medal (which she is wearing in the picture I posted)....I think she wore it for 2 days straight- I was able to convince her to take it off before she went to bed.

First grade continues to go well for Taylor- she is really enjoying it! She recently began having regular spelling tests, and loves writing in her journal at school and at home. She loves to write about anything and everything, and Rob and I just love to see all that she is learning.

The kids are looking forward to the holidays and all of the excitement that it brings. There are plans to go to the Nutcracker ballet, Christmas parades...and even a couple more races too! I love how busy the next couple of months will be!

So, love to all, and we wish you a happy and healthy holiday season. Thank you again for following Taylor's site and keeping up with her progress.

Love, Rob, Kim, Taylor, and Alex

December 18, 2009

Hi everyone! We are back from Gainesville- and everything continues to go well...

Taylor and I left early yesterday morning with suitcases packed...anticipating that we would be spending Thursday night in Gainesville so that they could remove her port first thing this morning. (Let me just say- she was not thrilled about that, but finally got in the car). Instead, we came home last night with suitcases untouched.....I'll start at the beginning :)

Taylor would have originally had her port out months ago- but with the couple of issues that came up (e.g., the abnormal cells after the final bone marrow biopsy...the relapse scare that prompted another bone marrow biopsy...), we weren't about to take the port out (and the doctors agreed). Once everything settled down, Rob took Taylor for a surgical consult and the surgeon suggested doing the surgery right before

Christmas break (to allow time to heal, no time away from school, etc.). So, the plan was to call in December and get this done! Since that time though, the surgeon has left Shands- so understandably, we needed to go for another surgical consult before another surgeon would take on her case...fair enough :) So, it worked out nicely to schedule that consult yesterday on the same day as her check-up with her hema- tology / oncology doctors at clinic. We met with the sur- geon...who was very nice...but explained that the operating schedule for Friday was booked, and that we would have to come back another day. Not a big deal in the scheme of things in our minds...So, Rob and I are figuring that out....Needless to say, Taylor was okay with that decision. We had some BIG talks over the past couple of days about this. In fact, she told the doctors yesterday that "January 12th is a good day for me- I'm not doing anything that day." (the funny thing is that the doctors didn't even bring up January 12th as an op- tion...)I'm so glad they can keep a straight face.

Taylor's doctors have told us that it is common for kids to be upset about removing their "buddy." It's been her lifeline for the past 3 years, and all of us have built it up for the past 3 years (e.g., "your buddy will help you! you won't get any pokes for blood draws or medicine!") In fact, they even give the kids their buddy (cleaned up of course!) in a glass jar after surgery. Taylor is excited about this. She would like "buddy" to stay with her in her room...and said she'd like to decorate the jar so buddy has a nice place to live....I'm sure at some point buddy will end up in the back of the closet and forgot- ten- but I guess we have to let her do that on her own terms. It is very interesting though.

So- for other good news- her counts looked fine, and all in acceptable ranges. The machine had some trouble reading her platelets, so the lab tech looked at them, but the reading showed somewhere between 156 and 177 which her doctors were fine with. It is always such a relief to hear their comfort level. I continually pray for acceptance of any news I am about to hear when she gets her counts checked, but I am human...and I still feel just sick while we're waiting (especially if it is taking a long time at the lab). Being at Shands reminds me to count our blessings every day, and that Taylor is here with us. While we were at clinic, we stopped by to see Taylor's infusion nurses (the ones that administered her chemo during treatment), and walking through the halls can just be surreal...there are so many children in the various stages of treatment, and the flash backs of being at that part of treatment come racing back to you...It just breaks your heart to know that there are so many families on this journey right now. It reminds me how amazing Taylor's doctors are- they are truly doing God's work and just work relentlessly to save these children. When I gave Dr. Slayton his Christmas Card yesterday...what I wanted to really say was "Thank You for another Christmas."

After clinic, Taylor and I spent some time having a picnic at the museum by the Butterfly Rainforest...and then of course spent some time with the butterflies! She really enjoys the rainforest, and was thrilled that a butterfly landed on her jacket. It is a very peaceful place to visit, and it was just a nice way to end the day. We've made several trips there over the past few years, and if a quick visit there helps to calm her anxiety about having to go to Gainesville- I'm okay with that. And while I had a list of 20 things on my mind about what I could get accomplished in Tallahassee if I "got back right away," I reminded myself to slow down, take a deep breath, and just enjoy the moment with my daughter...who handles these very stressful visits with such grace.

So, clinic was good, and our travels were safe. Many thanks to Grandma, Grandpa, and Aunt Debbie who made sure that Alex got to and from school and could have a "special sleep-over" last night while Mommy and Taylor were gone. Rob has been gone the past few days (in Buffalo, NY), so my parents and sister continue to be a God-send in helping to keep everything going (and some sort of schedule going for the girls!) Rob has been in Buffalo for a funeral for Uncle Jack's brother...who passed away a week ago today from cancer. Please keep Jack and his family in your prayers, as they have been amazing caretakers to his brother Dick, and have now had to endure the pain of losing him to this awful disease. It doesn't make sense (to us), but it is comforting to know that Dick is now in heaven and not in any more pain.

So, this year...when we walk in Relay, we will walk for all of our loved ones who are now in heaven...and we walk for all of those survivors still here with us. It feels like we all hear of new cases too often...Prayers and thoughts go out to De-anna (a friend's stepmother recently diagnosed with breast cancer), and to 2 new cases of little ones that were recently diagnosed (Hayley from Tallahassee www.caringbridge.org/visit/hayleyhart), and Brock from Oklahoma (related to a friend at work www.caringbridge.org/visit/brockhart). I read their postings, and pray for healing every day, but I know that extra prayers are always appreciated.

On a holiday note, our days have been filled with a lot of fun activities...there have been lots of fun holiday parties, we've gone to the Nutcracker Ballet (and the Ballerina breakfast!), a trip through the live Nativity with Grandma and Grandpa, the girls have been busy with their school and dance activities, and we have the Jingle Bell Run and Christmas parade this weekend! Life is good, and daily craziness feels like a blessing (when we stop to remember it that way).

Thank you to all of you- for praying for Taylor, for following this journey...for everything. If I don't say it enough- know how much we appreciate all of your kind words, notes, and support. In fact, I haven't had the chance to post about Taylor's friend Amelia who recently cut her hair and donated it to Locks of Love in honor of Taylor...what a wonderful thing to do at 6 years old! (Thank you Anoush and Steve!) Taylor adores Amelia, and Taylor keeps telling me that when her hair grows long enough, she's going to donate some too!

So, we send our love and Christmas wishes to all of you. Remember to hold your family close and hug them a little tighter this holiday season. We hope all of you have a very Merry Christmas, and we'll keep you posted on Taylor's progress!

Love, Rob, Kim, Taylor, and Alex

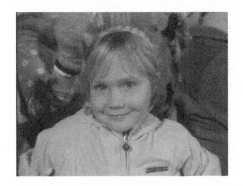

2010

Hello everyone! I know it has been awhile since I've updated, so let me start by saying that we hope that everyone had a wonderful holiday season, and that the New Year is going well...

Things here are going very normal, which is nice. From the picture on the front page, I'm sure you can tell that the girls are very excited about a new member of the family at Grandma and Grandpa's house! "Tramp" the puppy (so far- that's his name...as in "Lady and the Tramp") is 8 weeks old and is just adorable...As you can imagine, getting the girls to leave Grandma and Grandpa's house last night was quite the challenge....we convinced them that they would see Tramp again very soon.

Taylor is doing well and had her January visits with her pediatrician here locally. Her blood counts came back in normal ranges- in fact, her WBC was 6.2 (which is the highest we've ever seen it), so we continue to be thankful for God's blessings in her continued progress. Our next trip to Gainesville will include Taylor's surgery to remove her port (i.e., this is the "trip we do not speak of")- as she is still not thrilled about it- but it has to be done. She is coming up on 1 year of being done with chemo (Wow!), and it's time for buddy to come out. I think she is coming to terms with it, but even if she's not completely there, we'll continue to work through it with her. She has told us that she "hates her visits to Shands more than anything in this world...." We know that she's just scared, and by the way- she's allowed to be, so while my heart breaks for her- someday she will understand it was all necessary and all in her best interest.

All in all though, life is wonderful- busy, but wonderful. The girls continue to do well in school, and are looking forward to some exciting things....like the Daddy / Daughter dance! So, we will update again soon, and just ask for your prayers as Taylor comes to terms with her next surgery.

Love to all, and thank you again for following Taylor....

Love, Rob, Kim, Taylor, and Alex

February 16, 2010

Big milestone....Taylor had her surgery this past Friday to take out her "buddy."

She did great...and we now have buddy in a jar...I'll admit- it was kind of weird to think that it has been inside her for 3 years now....wow...it's been quite the journey!

We started off with a trip to clinic on Thursday, and I can't explain how good it feels for the doctor to come in smiling, hug you, and tell you "Kim, her counts look perfect." Dr. Slayton feels good with her progress, and said that the next step is to do an echocardiogram during her next visit. (Basically- an ultrasound of her heart to see how things are going). He explained that they like to do this one-year post-chemo to check on her heart. You may remember that when we were in the 'delayed intensification' phase of treatment (about 6 months into it)- the doctors did a baseline echocardiogram prior to administering some of the specific types of chemo (that had a potential side effect of heart damage). So, now it is just time to do a comparison. We have faith that everything will continue to be fine.

So, the Thursday clinic visit went well, and then the four of us went together on Friday for Taylor's surgery. The one tough part was that her surgery got pushed back a few hours, and she was pretty hungry while we waited (because she wasn't allowed to eat prior to surgery), but it is what it is....and she pushed through just fine. Recovery went fine- little bit of nausea, but some Zofran helped that subside. Alex was a very good nurse to Taylor....rubbing her back afterwards, bringing her Gatorade, and just telling her that she would be fine. And then of course- there was the thing that kept Taylor distracted through a lot of this....we headed to Disney for the weekend to celebrate. It was a nice weekend together, and then the kids were able to relax with Daddy on Monday (since school was out for Teacher Planning day). So, all in all- we're doing good, and just so proud of Taylor for getting through all of this.

She asked me if this was the "last time she was going to have to take sleepy juice," and we told her "yes." She was happy. I think she also misunderstood and thought that she wouldn't have to go to Gainesville anymore for checkups....so we've had that discussion as well- but I told her that the checkups will start to get less frequent....that made it a little better!

So, we'll keep everyone posted on our next trip to Shands, and thank you again for following Taylor and for your prayers....she has passed yet another milestone!

Love, Rob, Kim, Taylor, and Alex

April 5, 2010

We hope that everyone had a Happy Easter! Things continue to go well in the Koegel household...(hence our lack of updates to the site...which is a good thing I guess!) We had a wonderful Easter, and it was a perfect ending to the kids' Spring Break last week. Over Spring Break, we had a chance to spend time in Orlando and visit with friends and family. The kids got in lots of swim time (they were like fish!), and spent some time at Disney too (including a Yankees / Braves Spring Training game)...so it was a fun time. We spent Easter at Grandma and Grandpa's house- and there was a fun surprise of a Slip N' Slide when we got to their house! You can imagine the fun we all had while Easter dinner was cooking....it was truly some of the most fun we've had on Easter in a while!

Today- it was back to work and back to school- I think all of us were a bit tired, but we made it through! We are looking ahead to a busy week, including a trip to Shands for Taylor. She'll have a check-up on Thursday that includes an echocardiogram to verify that all is fine with her heart (1-year post-chemo). We have faith that all is fine, but this is just a standard test that the doctors do to help ensure that the chemotherapy did not adversely affect her heart.

Taylor has been doing great. School and her activities are going well. She seems to be growing up so fast, and we are constantly reminded of how aware she is of everything now. She does not enjoy her trips to Shands, and we are hopeful that these will become less frequent- but until then, it is just something we help her deal with. She doesn't throw a fit....she simply tolerates the trips, but she isn't afraid to tell you how much she hates going! It has also been interesting as we approach this year's Relay for Life. We will be participating, but I will admit that to date- we were a bit touch and go as we tried to get a sense of how Taylor felt about participating. She really wants to go, but has asked that no one "make a big deal" about how she had cancer....It is insightful to hear your 6-year-old say that to you....she really just wants to be a kid and go enjoy being at Relay...but not be part of the focus. So, with that in mind- we are now in "Relay" mode as we try to reach our goal of $1,000. Will it be our last year at Relay? I don't think so- possibly our last year as "Team Princess Taylor,"- we'll look to Taylor and her comfort level to participate as a team in the future....but this is a cause that Rob and I will continue to participate in at some level because we know it is such an important

cause. Rob and I continue to be thankful for the research and treatments that have come about as a result of the fundraising efforts of the American Cancer Society. When I think about the life-saving protocols that were available to Taylor, and the educational programs that the American Cancer Society has provided us as part of this experience- we are just so appreciative.

So, we'd ask you to consider pledging your support to Team Princess Taylor (http://main.acsevents.org/goto/teamprincesstaylor). Whether you would like to join the team or prefer

to donate, every bit helps in this fight for hope...Like I say on our team website:

"We relay for Taylor, and we relay for so many others that have battled, are battling, and may battle this awful disease...We relay for their caregivers...We relay for everyone who has waited for test results, feared relapse, endured chemotherapy, asked "why me?", and for those that may have to hear that news someday."

The event is Friday, May 14th...so if you are in the Tallahassee area, come out and walk with us!!!

We'll keep everyone posted on Taylor's clinic visit this week and her continued progress. Love to all....

Love, Rob, Kim, Taylor, and Alex

May 14, 2010

Hello to everyone- Here we are already to May 14th! Tonight is the Relay for Life and Team Princess Taylor is ready to go! (http://main.acsevents.org/goto/teamprincesstaylor).

Thank you to everyone who is coming out to walk tonight or has supported our efforts for this cause.

I know that I mentioned in my last post that we had chosen to slightly "downplay" the focus on Relay this year per Taylor's request...well, things have changed a bit, and she is now in planning mode. When I mentioned to her on Wednesday that the Relay was almost here, she told me "Well, I've decided that I want our theme to be "Christmas." I told her that we only had 2 days left...and that I wasn't sure what the overall theme was, but that I would check. She then told me

"I don't care what the overall theme is...why can't ours just be "Christmas?" (the beauty of being 6 years old....) So then, ironically, I check the overall theme yesterday- and the theme is "Birthdays Around the World."

One of my coworkers reminded me that there isn't a more important birthday than Jesus' birthday....Yep, she's right....So, out of the mouth of babes comes an innocent request for a Christmas theme, and somehow we tie it all together in the end.

So- we'll see what we can pull together in terms of some basic Christmas decorations today :)

So, Relay has kept us busy this week, and life overall continues to busy and normal- so that makes us happy. School is going well- hard to believe that Taylor is wrapping up 1st grade and will be a 2nd grader before we know it!

Taylor's visits to Shands continue to be every other month, and during her April visit, her doctors told Rob that they are fine with us not going to see our local pediatrician on the "off" months....which means we just cut her visits in half! She'll have her next visit to Shands in June, at which time I guess they will also go over any echocardiogram results with us, but other than that- we are assuming that regular visits should just include bloodwork / counts check and a general check-up by the doctors. Rob mentioned to me that the doctors seemed very pleased about her progress and that she was at the 1-year mark with being done with chemo (when she was there in April). He told me that their reaction made him feel like the 1-year mark was a significant milestone. We hope it is- and we never forget that her doctors have done so much to get her where she is today. We will always worry, but just continue to pray for continued health, patience, understanding....and normalcy for Taylor.

As I close out this post, I just wanted to thank everyone again for following Taylor's journey. Unfortunately, we hear of too many cases of new little ones being diagnosed with cancer, and when I hear their stories- it takes me back to January of 2007 and how we had such an outpouring of support from everyone. Recently, Trent, a Kindergartner at Taylor's school was diagnosed, and is currently receiving treatment in Texas. We'll be walking tonight for Taylor, Trent, and so many others....

Love to all, and we'll keep you posted on Taylor's upcoming visit.

Love, Rob, Kim, Taylor, and Alex

August 31, 2010

Hello everyone! Yes, it has been a long time since an update- which in a way is a very positive thing! Taylor continues to do great, and is now in 2nd grade- wow!

When I looked at Taylor and Alex in their 'first day of school' pictures, it just struck me at how fast they are growing up. On days like that, it feels like time flies....and then I think back to Taylor's treatment, and I remember how it felt like time was crawling- but day by day, we put another day between us and a lot of those tough times...and just remember to be thankful for her progress.

The girls have been doing great- a great summer with lots to keep them busy. Taylor also received good news in June during her trip to Shands regarding the frequency of her visits. We now only have to travel to Shands every 4 months. She does need to have blood counts at the 2-month mark (and see her pediatrician here locally)- but little by little, and year by year- the visits will become less frequent. She hit the 2-month mark last week- and had her blood counts done here- and they were great- higher than they've ever been. And yes...we still have the sigh of relief and the prayer of thanks that come when they call you with the results. We'll head to Shands in October for her next visit.

So life is feeling busy, but good- looking ahead to a Fall filled with school, activities, and football....and seeing who wins the Clemson / FSU game :) Taylor is starting soccer, and is very excited...Her daddy has been practicing with her.

I've also been thinking a lot about the "right time" to wrap up the updates to our Caring Bridge site. It has been such a blessing to have this site- it was a lifesaver during treatment- especially when things were changing so dramatically- day to day- or I needed a venue to get all of my feelings out...and we thank all of you for your continued support and postings- this site helped us more than I can ever explain. And while I know this journey doesn't end, Rob and I pray that we are through the worst of it, and that all of this becomes a distant memory for Taylor. As Taylor gets older- and I don't know what the right time will be- these journal entries will help us explain so much to her.

Had we not written it all down....there would be no way to recall the various emotions going on at the time.

So- we'll figure that out...and know that while we don't up- date as frequently as we used to, we have appreciated your prayers and support over the past 3 years, and we look for- ward to keeping everyone posted on Taylor as she continues to progress and amaze her Daddy and me.

Love to all, and we hope that all is going well.

Love, Rob, Kim, Taylor, and Alex

Kim Koegel

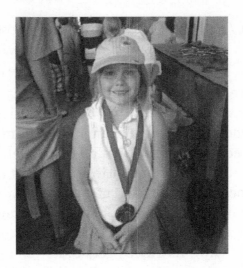

2011

We hope that everyone had a wonderful Easter! It is hard to believe that another Spring is here and that Taylor has passed the 2-year mark since her treatment wrapped in March 2009. She and Rob traveled to Gainesville the week before last for her 2-year check-up, and her lab work was all in normal ranges. Such a blessing, and such a reminder of how God continues to bless us each and every day. Her visits have now been spread out so that she only has to visit Shands every 3 months....so her next visit will be in July.

While it has been awhile since we've updated the site, life continues to be full of things that I wish I took time to journal about every day. Sometimes I wonder where the past 7 years(almost 8 years!) have gone! The girls are growing bigger every day, and are keeping busy with their activities. Taylor has really loved soccer and Brownies, and Alex loves dance class. It's hard to believe that Taylor will soon be a 3rd grader and that Alex will be in Kindergarten in just a few short months! Spring brings with it dance recitals, pre-school graduation, soccer games, school musicals, and Taylor's First Communion at church. Taylor has also asked to have Team Princess Taylor at Relay for Life again this year....It makes me smile...because as much as she sometimes says she is getting "too old for princesses," she insisted on keeping the team name the same.

We would love for you to come walk with us- even just for a lap or two! Relay is Friday night, May 13th...Visit the Team Princess Taylor site at http://main.acsevents.org/

goto/teamprincesstaylor and think about joining us for the evening...it is quite amazing.

We are doing a "superhero" theme...so like I say on the Relay site- get out your superhero cape (or your Wonder Woman boots)- and let's get walking!

All in all, things continue to go well, and we are just grateful for Taylor's continued progress. She asks a lot of questions now about Cancer, the procedures, and the medicines she had to take. Through all of her questions and our answers, she keeps an enduring faith that God has a reason for all of this, and that someday when we are all in Heaven...we will know the answer then. It has been the answer we have given her and Alex for all of the tough things that happen in life, and is something that Rob and I truly believe...I know it has gotten me through the past 4 years....

I am going to sign off for now, but do hope that everyone is doing well. Thank you for continuing to check in on Miss Taylor...she continues to amaze us.

Love, Kim, Rob, Taylor, and Alex

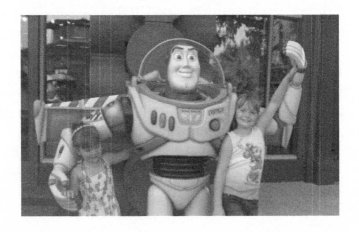

TEN YEARS LATER...

January 19, 2017

Ten years ago today, our life took an unexpected turn. It is hard to believe it was ten years ago today that Taylor was transported to Shands and hospitalized for what the doctors suspected to be Leukemia...only to confirm on January 20th that it absolutely was Leukemia-specifically Acute Lymphoblastic Leukemia (ALL). There are some dates you never forget, no matter how long ago something happened.

Fast forward ten years later...and you are standing with us tonight on the sidelines of Taylor's middle school soccer game ....the first game of her 8th grade season...watching her play an amazing game and helping her team secure a win. I probably cheered a little louder than I needed to tonight- I often do- but deep down inside I was cheering for so much more than just a soccer game. Ten years ago I watched a little girl hanging on to life...Tonight I watched my teenager run up and down a field more times than I could count- with what seemed like endless energy. What a different place we are in today.

The past ten years have continued to give us balanced perspective of what is most important in our lives. We have had highs and lows, good health and a couple of scares here and there- but through it all, we have had an amazing network of family and friends to see us through. I've also consciously tried to remember to not overlook "the little things" going on in life...knowing that someday I will look back and remember that "all of those little things were really the big things" and are making such great memories.

Taylor doesn't know what today is...or tomorrow is...or that those dates should mean anything to her- and I am okay with that. Cancer did not define her. I do think it shaped her, but it does not define her. I look at her now and see a strong-willed, beautiful 13-year-old who has goals of becoming a doctor one day. If you asked her, she would probably define herself as a soccer player...a runner...a middle schooler...a teenager...but Cancer would never enter the conversation. I thank God regularly that she was so young when she went through treatment. Her memories of that time in her life are a bit blurry...and that is okay. The less she has to remember about any of it, the better. Having said that, she is older now, and she understands the gravity of her annual check-ups and she is absolutely listening to every word the doctors say...she is absolutely in tune with what is going on around her and the importance of living healthy, staying active, and making good choices.

Several people have mentioned to me over the years that I should have written a book about the blogs we kept during that time- and while I have waited a long time to get it started- it isn't out of the question yet. I do know that I would title it "Faith, Love, and Applesauce" as I have considered in the past that these were the three most important things that got us through that time in our life. I truly believe that our Faith grew leaps and bounds with each day- knowing that God would give us the strength as we made this journey....Love was abundant from our family, friends...and even total strangers who reached out to us to express support and offer prayers. We can't thank everyone enough for the support you showed us. And finally- Applesauce. I used to joke that we should have purchased stock in Mott's Applesauce. Taylor will not eat applesauce to this day- as she ate it / used it every day for almost 3 years to swallow her medicine...I get if she's a little over it.

So thank you for reading this update tonight- We are so

thankful for all of you and your ongoing support and love for our family.

Love, Rob, Kim, Taylor and Alex

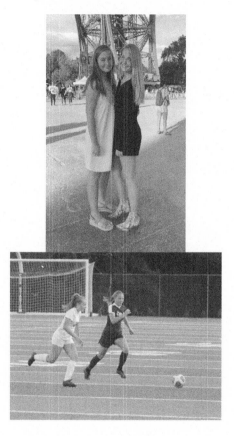